To my magnificent
husband, Ryan:
The butter to my bread,
the icing to my cake, and
the one who always makes
life more delicious.

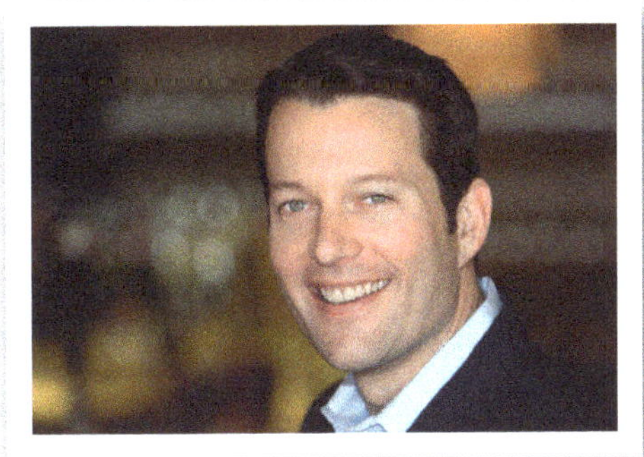

Paperback ISBN: 979-8-88526-408-2

Book design by Joe Hall and Natasha McCone, with invaluable contrubutions by Kate Bezak

FROM THE

Sticky Fingers Cooking®

SCHOOL

The Third Cookbook

BASIC TRAINING BAKING BOOT CAMP

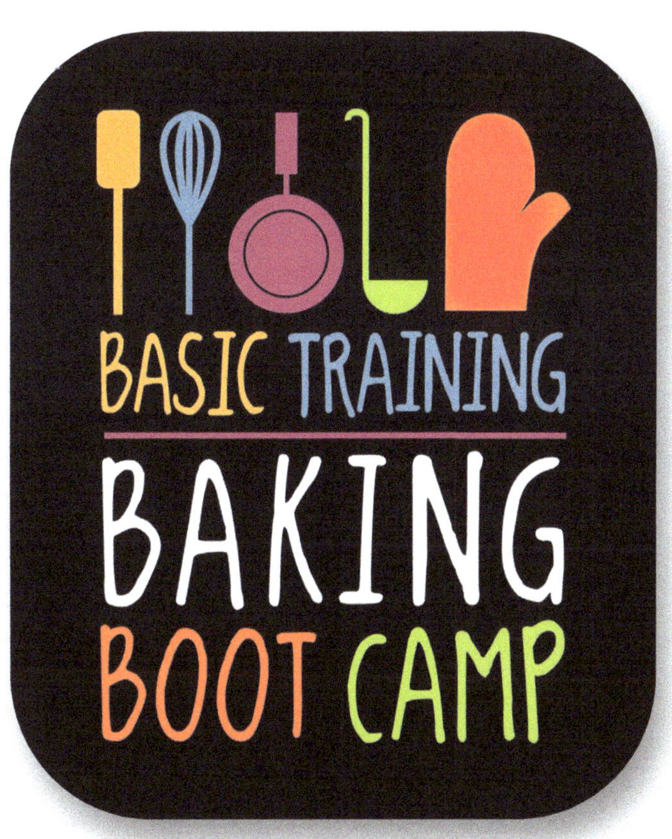

"This crostata tastes just like a basket of blackberries but like a million times better!"
- Patrick, age 8

"I am going to be a professional baker and took Sticky Fingers Cooking (classes) so I could also learn savory baking"
- Leila, age 6

"The cranberries in the compote really complement the pumpkin in the flapjacks."
- Benjamin, age 7

the Sticky Fingers Cooking® School

Sticky Fingers Cooking is an acclaimed mobile and online children's cooking school providing inspiring "hands-on" cooking classes to over 50,000 students since 2011. We recognize the value of fostering curiosity, independence, confidence, and development of essential, lifelong cooking skills through interactive and engaging culinary experiences.

We whisk together a sense of fun within all of our specially-developed, kid-friendly curriculum and in our over 800 proprietary recipes designed to expand children's skills and palates. We combine and connect our love of culinary arts with nutritional information, safe cooking skills, language, geography, math, science, and food history to help inspire and ignite a lifetime love of healthy cooking and adventurous eating that children relish.

"Mom, no offence but my breads are better than yours."
- Emily, age 7

"I would add grated beets again to get healthy stuff and still get to eat a doughnut!"
- Kai, age 8

"I love Sticky Fingers SO much I'm going to take classes until I go to college"
- Liam, age 10

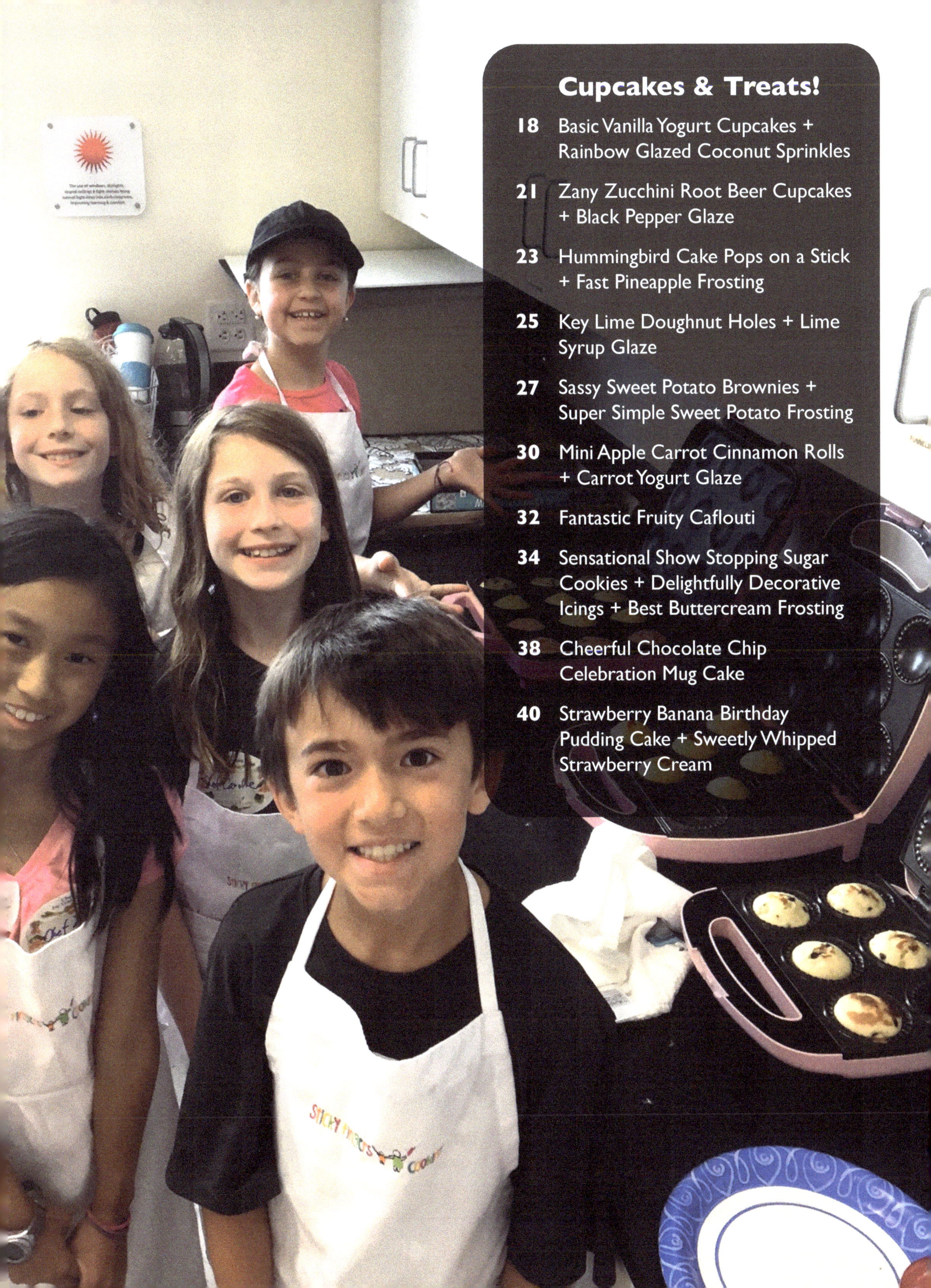

Cupcakes & Treats!

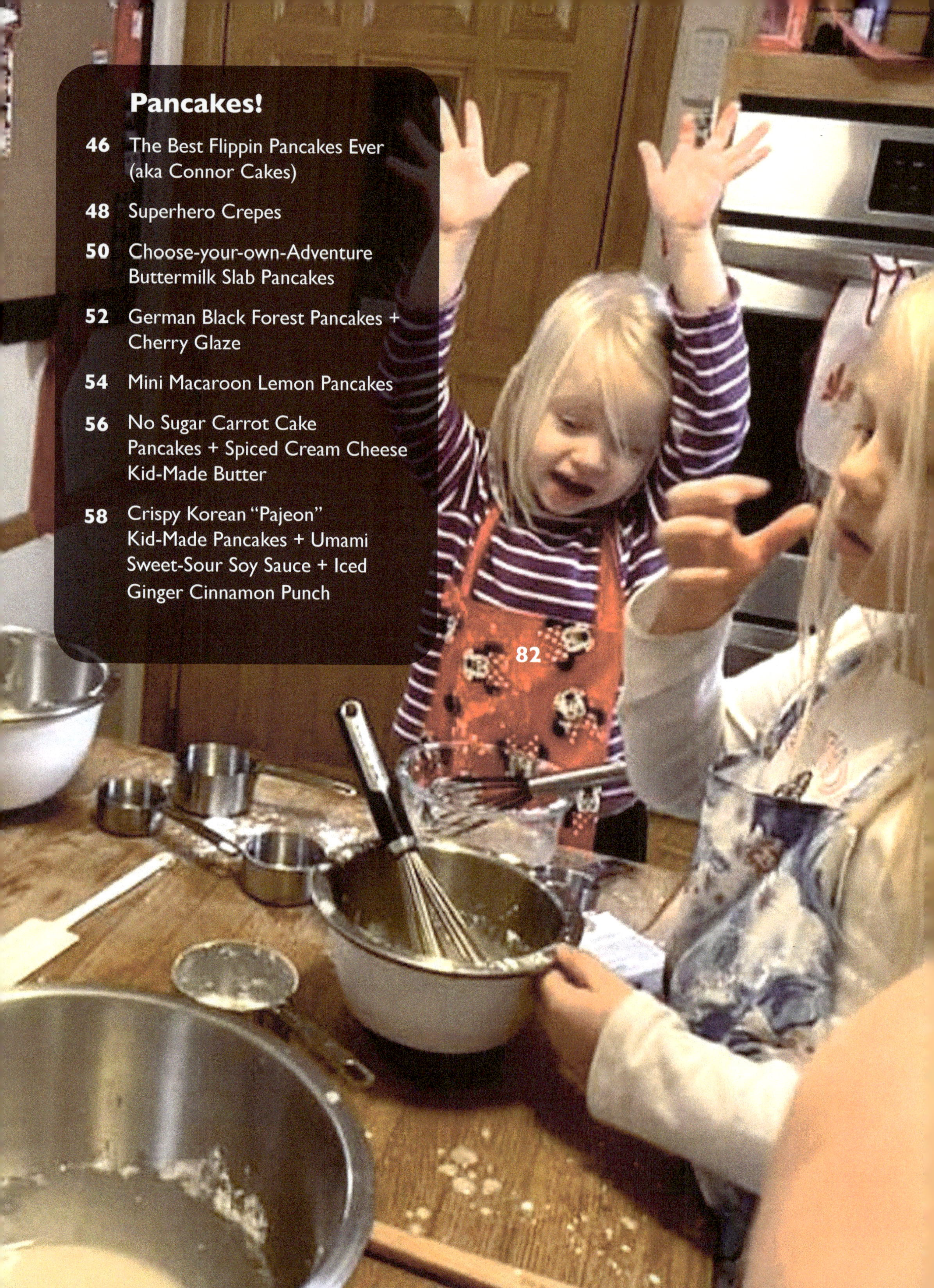

Pancakes!

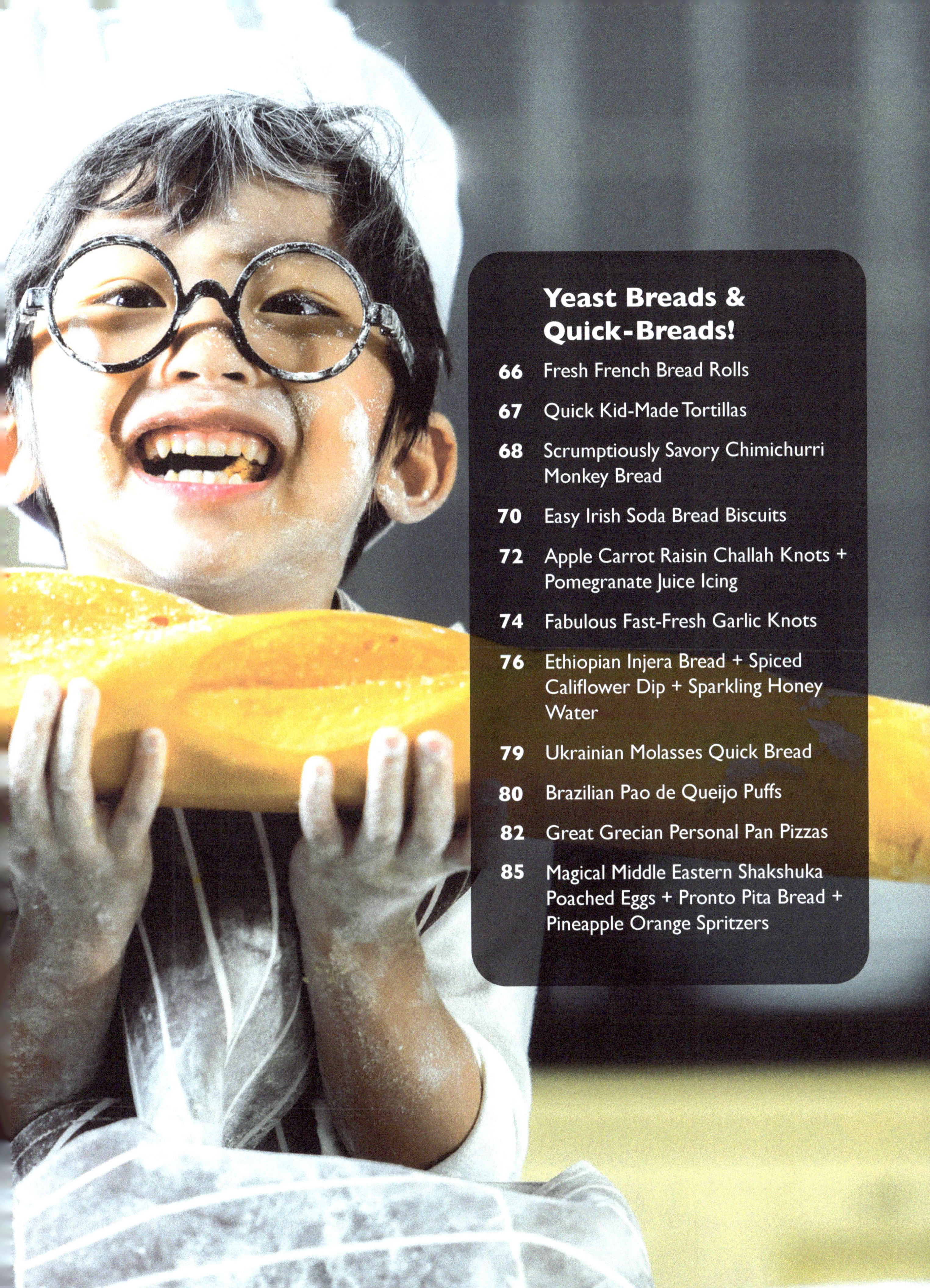

Yeast Breads & Quick-Breads!

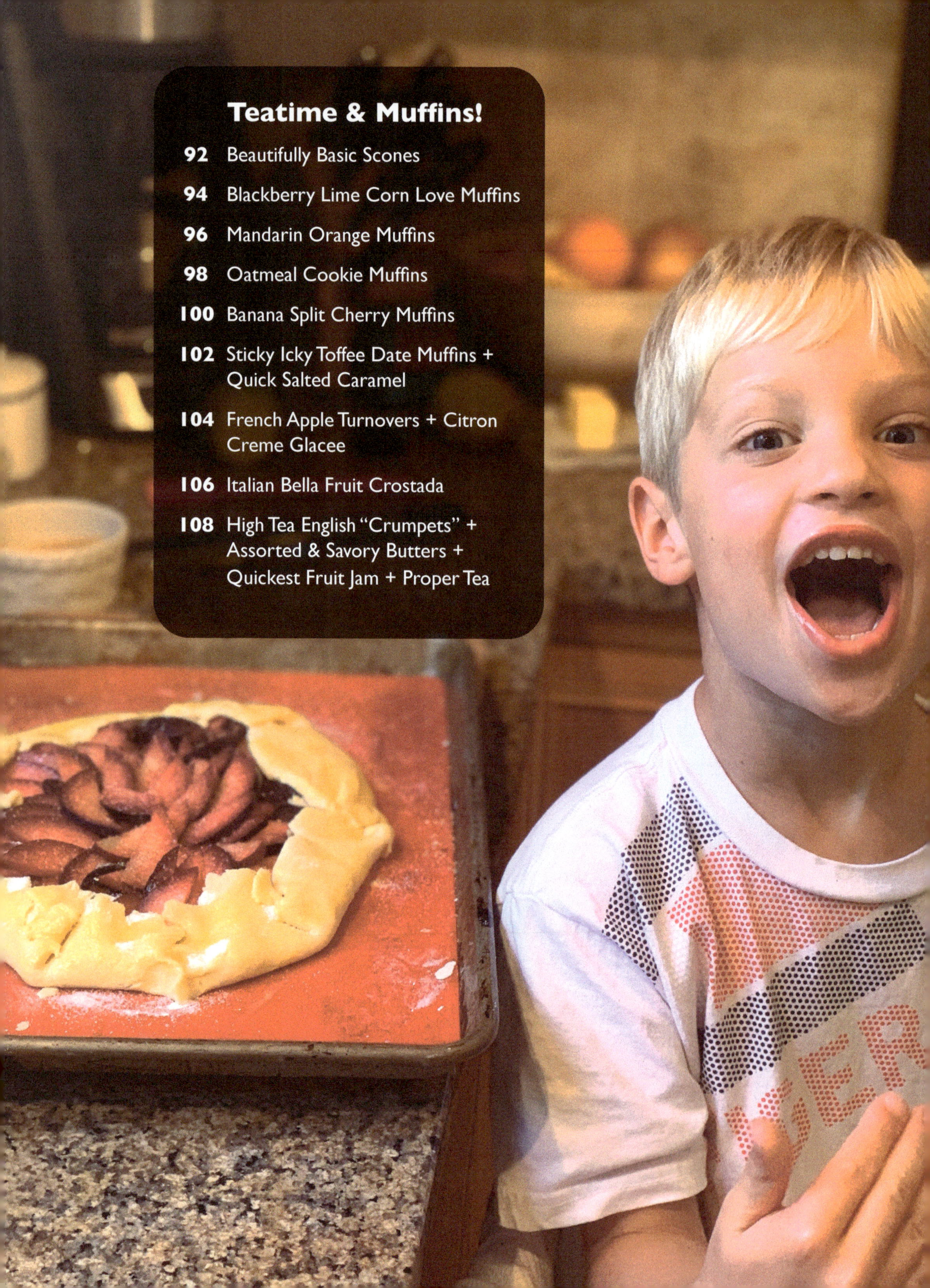

Teatime & Muffins!

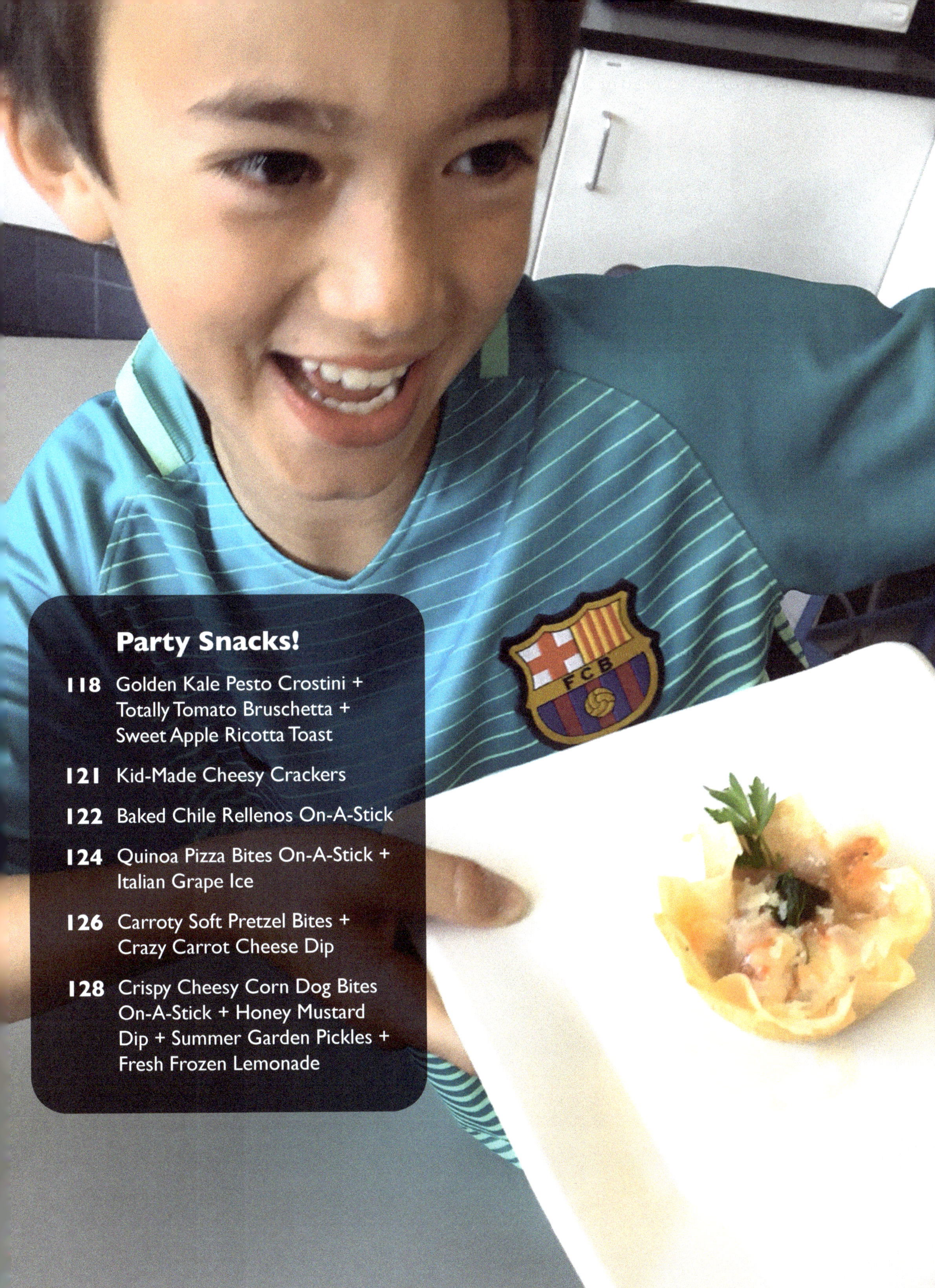

Party Snacks!

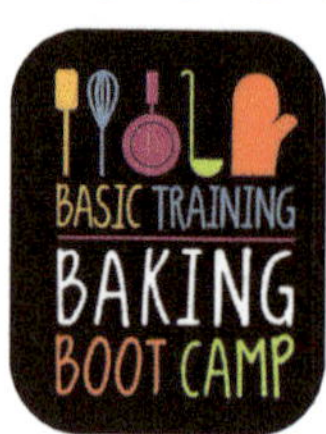

INTRODUCTION

Welcome to Sticky Fingers Cooking's Basic Training Baking Boot Camp

"If baking is any labor at all, it's a labor of love. A love that gets passed from generation to generation." *-Regina Brett*

From encouraging healthy eating to discovering hidden science, baking with your kids offers plenty of perks. Stir the flour mix, measure one cup of buttermilk, roll out the dough… Yes, all of these baking tasks help kids develop necessary academic, cognitive, and motor skills. While baking with your kids offers a wide variety of opportunities to learn and grow, it can provide a more robust and profound impact: connection and lifelong memories. The thing about baking is, it's never just baking.

Whether preparing bread, muffins, or crepes, my family and I always find ourselves chatting and smiling in the kitchen. Good food operates as its own language. The dialogue is endless. Baking is an opportunity to connect, create memories with your kids, learn lifelong skills, and, most importantly, "be" in the present moment. I hope this cookbook will give you a platform to explore baking with your family while being present with gratitude. You will find some historical family recipes sprinkled throughout to support this notion. I hope you discover your spark of creativity, rename these recipes as your own family recipes, and create your own "un-recipes", all while having conversations and memories with your kids that will last a lifetime.

It's beautiful to know that something as simple as baking together can bring so much love and connection to a family.

Learn, bake, love + share,

Erin Fletter, Food-Geek-In-Chief, Co-Founder Sticky Fingers Cooking

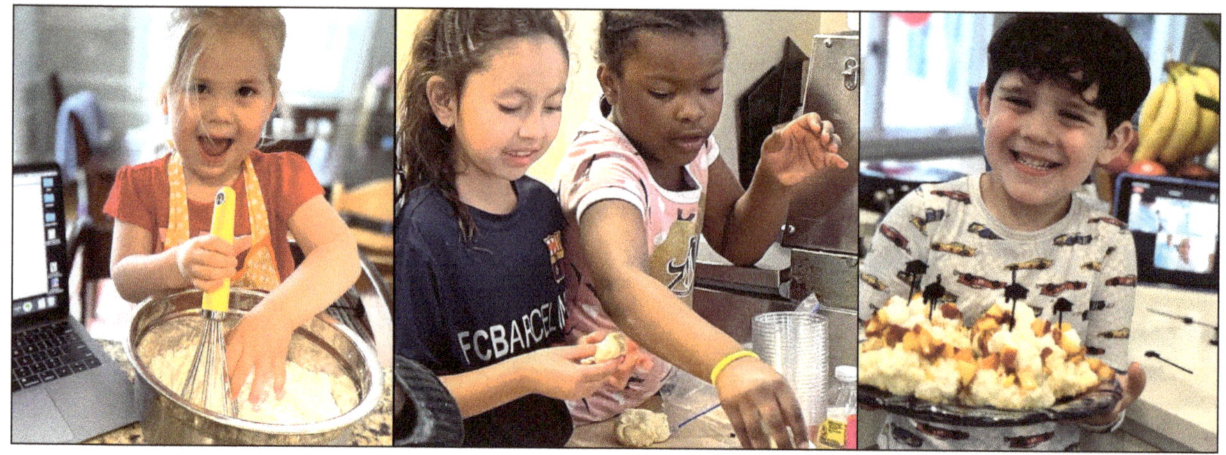

HOW TO USE THE COOKBOOK

Baking is one of the easiest ways to introduce kids to cooking, and what better way to approach baking than to empower kids to create their own recipes! In this unique cookbook, young chefs and their families have the opportunity to explore the wonderful world of baking - both sweet and savory. You and your young chefs will learn the foundations of baking and then use that knowledge to create your own special recipes that are sure to become family favorites in no time.

You'll notice *Baking Boot Camp* looks a little different than our previous two cookbooks, *Global Taste Buds* and *Farm to Table.* *Baking Boot Camp* is designed to amp up the fun in the kitchen and let kids' imaginations run wild. Each recipe section includes a **101 Junior Chef** recipe, which gently encourages you and your kids to play with different flavors and pairings to gain more confidence, and our advanced **201 Top Chef** recipes that provide your kids with opportunities for a full-meal experience. You'll be pleasantly surprised and impressed with what your kids can bake when they're the chefs!

As a cooking school we have always said, "if kids make it, they'll eat it." We have stood by this motto since our inception in 2011, and we have tens of thousands of our students to back up that claim. However, we would slightly amend our motto to this: "if kids decide what they make, they'll eat it." In addition to including over 70 recipes, this cookbook takes a unique approach to baking with kids by empowering them to create their own, unique "un-recipes" for frostings, butters, calzones, and more! Each recipe section includes a visual guide to help your kids on their way to confectionary adventure. Our hope is that this style of cookbook will inspire creativity in the kitchen and foster a sense of empowerment, all the while still having fun, of course! Baking, just like cooking, is meant to be fun.

Baking is also a science, where temperature, measurement, and proportion all play key roles in achieving a beautiful bake, but that can make baking with allergies more difficult. We understand the importance of accommodating allergies as we have taught countless kids' cooking classes and accommodated ANY and ALL allergies. We have included information to enable people with gluten, dairy, and/or egg allergies enjoy our delicious recipes without worry … so you and your kids can bake to your heart's delight!

There is nothing quite like baking in the kitchen with your family. Baking is nostalgic and can bring back childhood memories with a simple whiff of cinnamon or vanilla. Flipping through a favorite family cookbook and seeing all your handwritten recipe notes can also bring those memories flooding back, so please don't be afraid to mark up and write notes all over this cookbook. That's what it's there for—to invite you to create your own family memories. With a pinch of laughter and a heap of love, we wish you and your family happy and healthy baking!

QUICK CONVERSIONS!

The measurements in baking can be intimidating but have no fear! Use this page to easily figure out your baking conversions.

1 tablespoon	3 teaspoons
6 teaspoons	2 tablespoons

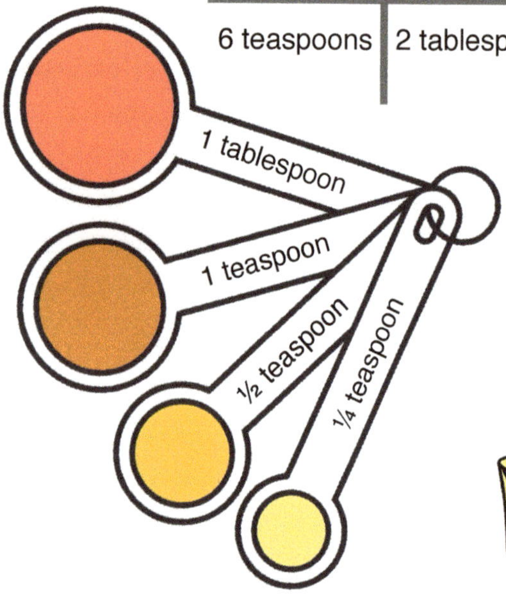

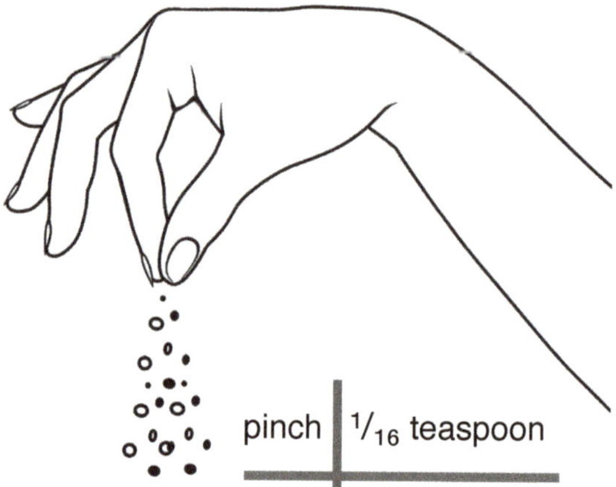

pinch	$^1/_{16}$ teaspoon
dash	⅛ teaspoon

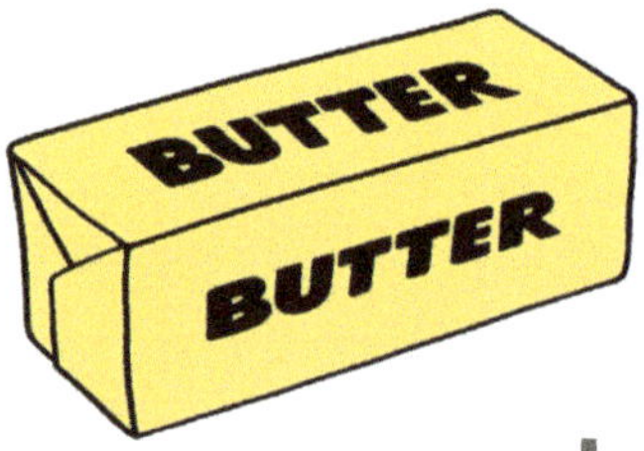

½ stick	¼ cup	4 tablespoons
1 stick	½ cup	8 tablespoons
2 sticks	1 cup	16 tablespoons

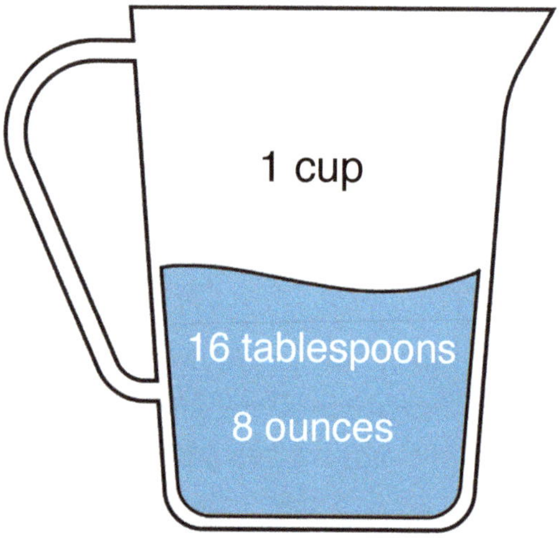

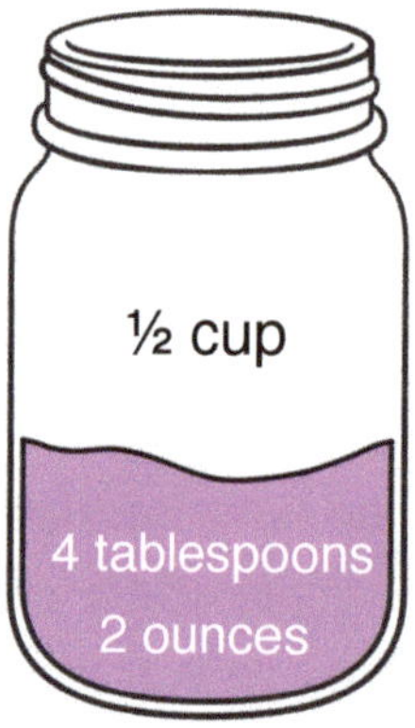

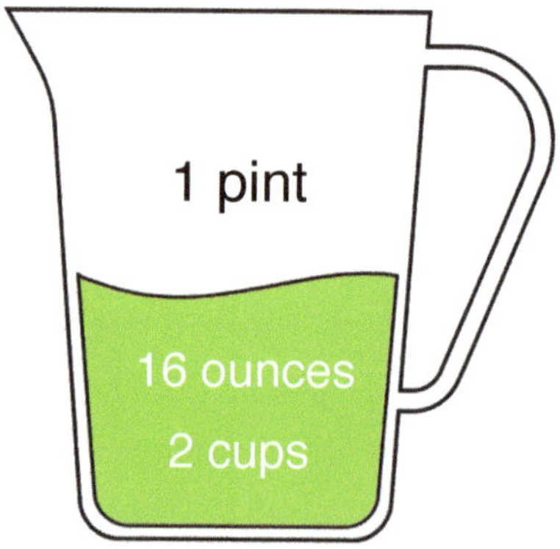

MEASURING: Baking is a science! When measuring sugar or flour, use the back of a butter knife to level the top and get an exact measurement.

ALLERGY ALERT!

Those Sneaky Allergens…!

Did you know common allergens (gluten, dairy, egg) like to hide in everyday products and ingredients? They just might go by a different name! When baking for someone who has an allergy, it's important to be aware of those sneaky allergens in disguise.

Baking Dairy-Free

Find your favorite non-dairy milk: Coconut, almond, oat, rice, or soy make for great 1:1 substitutions.

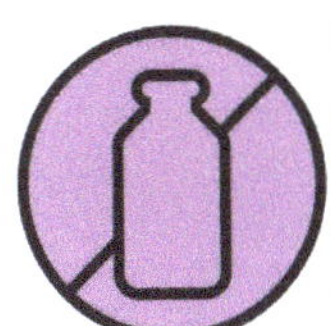

Buttermilk Substitution: Mix 1 tablespoon of lemon juice with 1 cup of non-dairy milk and let sit to curdle, which is what you want!

Cream Substitution: Soak cashews in water overnight and purèe the next day. Use a handheld mixer to whip the purèe into a thick, luscious cream!

Baking Gluten-Free

A 1:1 gluten-free flour blend is your best friend! Be sure to select a blend already containing xanthan gum.

Double check that your baking soda and powder are fresh.

Mix your doughs and batters longer than you would normally.

Let your doughs and batters take a longer nap. A good rule is to let them rest for at least 30 minutes.

Most important tip: forget perfection!

Baking Egg-Free

Aquafaba (the liquid leftover from cooked chickpeas or from a can of chickpeas):

3 tablespoons of aquafaba = 1 whole egg

2 tablespoons of aquafaba = 1 egg white

Substitute With Seeds:

Soak 2 tablespoons of chia seeds in 5 tablespoons of water for 5 to 8 minutes

Soak 1 tablespoon of ground chia or flaxseeds in 3 tablespoons of water for 5 minutes or until fully absorbed and thickened

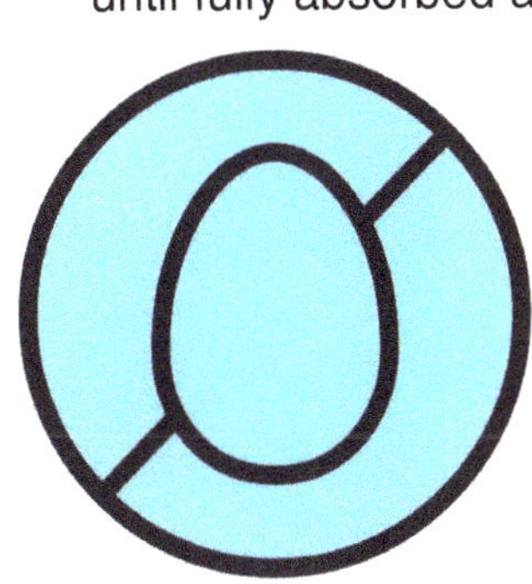

For pancakes/waffles, muffins, and quick sweet breads:

¼ cup of unsweetened applesauce or mashed banana

For brownies, cookies, quick breads, and cakes:

¼ cup of purèed silken tofu

For muffins, cakes, and cupcakes:

¼ cup of yogurt or buttermilk

For light and airy baked goods:

1 teaspoon of baking soda with 1 tablespoon of vinegar

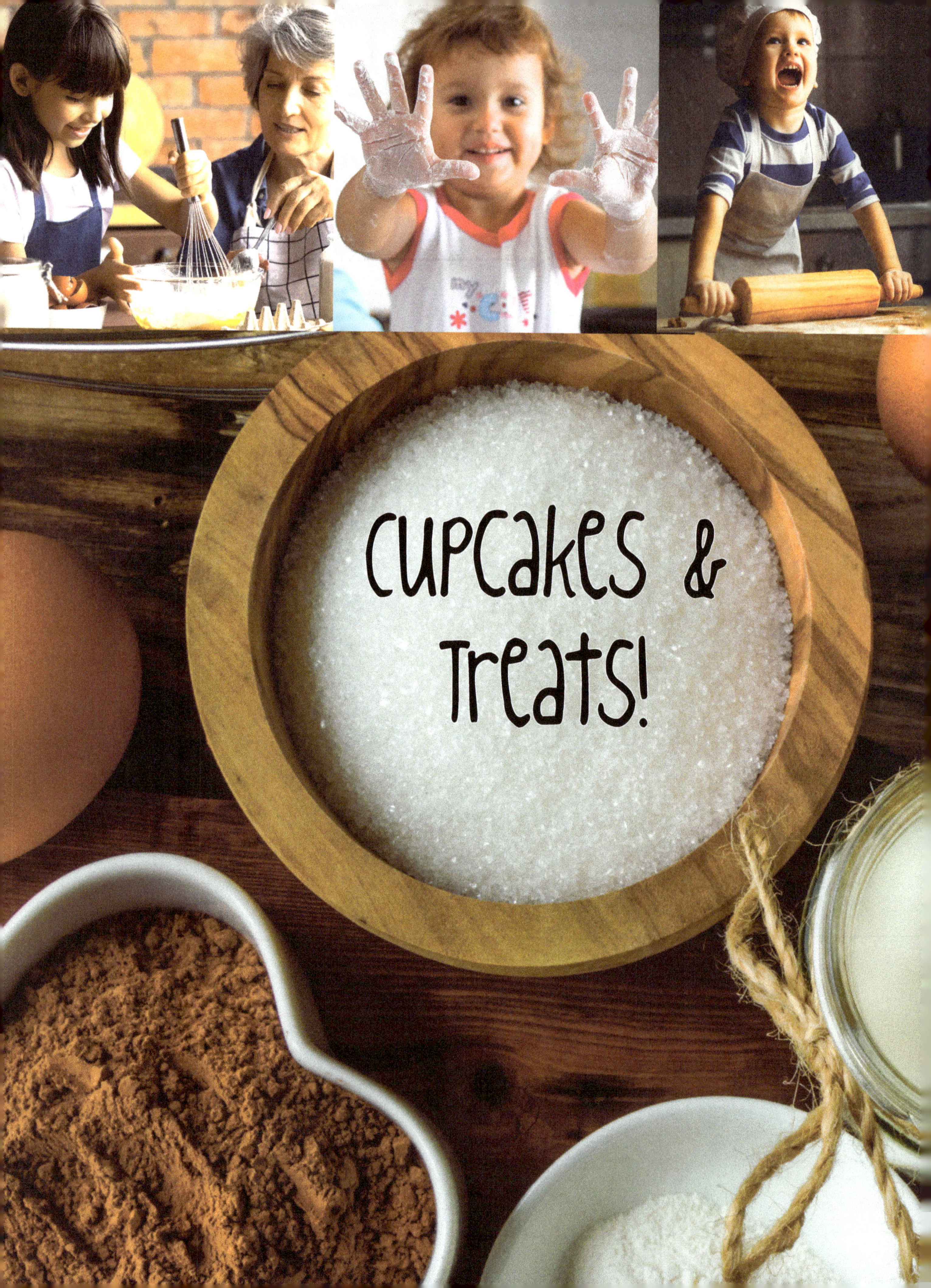

Cupcakes & Treats!

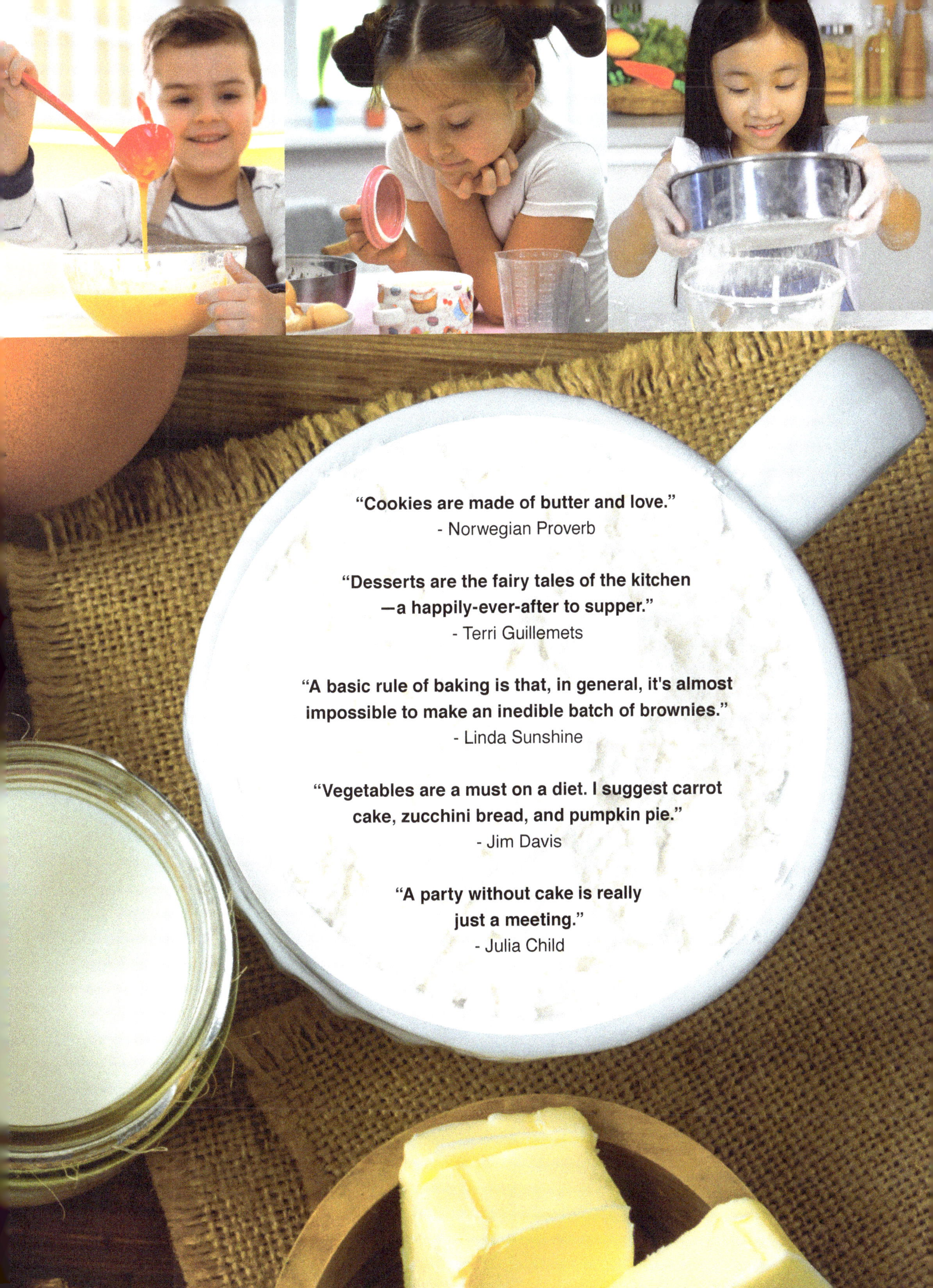
"Cookies are made of butter and love."
- Norwegian Proverb
"Desserts are the fairy tales of the kitchen
—a happily-ever-after to supper."
- Terri Guillemets
"A basic rule of baking is that, in general, it's almost
impossible to make an inedible batch of brownies."
- Linda Sunshine
"Vegetables are a must on a diet. I suggest carrot
cake, zucchini bread, and pumpkin pie."
- Jim Davis
"A party without cake is really
just a meeting."
- Julia Child

Basic Vanilla Yogurt Cupcakes + Rainbow Coconut Sprinkles

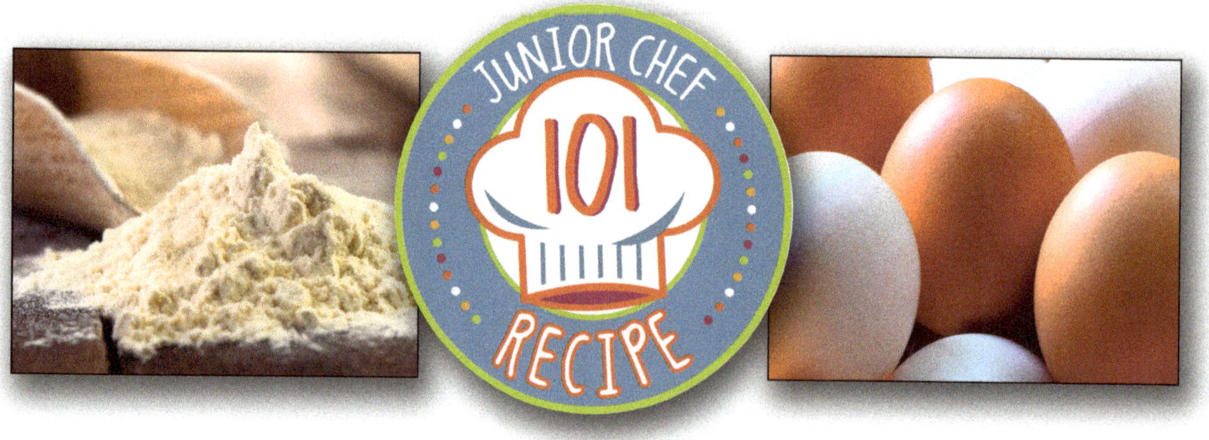

basic vanilla yogurt cupcakes

ingredients

- 1½ C all-purpose flour
- ½ tsp baking powder
- ¼ tsp baking soda
- ¼ tsp salt
- 1 C sugar
- 2 large eggs
- 1 C plain whole-milk yogurt
- 1 tsp vanilla extract
- ¼ C milk
- ½ C unsalted butter

preheat+measure+mix

Preheat your oven to 350 degrees F and line a muffin pan with paper liners. Mix together **1½ cups of flour, ½ teaspoon of baking powder, ¼ teaspoon of baking soda, ¼ teaspoon of salt,** and **1 cup of sugar** in a large bowl.

crack+stir

Crack **2 eggs** into a bowl and stir in **1 cup of yogurt, 1 teaspoon of vanilla extract, ¼ cup of milk,** and **½ cup of butter.**

whisk+pour+bake

Whisk the wet and dry ingredients together until smooth. Bake in your preheated oven for 16 to 18 minutes or until cooked through when tested with a toothpick.

rainbow coconut sprinkles

ingredients

fresh or frozen (thawed) raspberries
fresh or frozen (thawed) mangoes
roasted beets
raw carrots
spinach
radicchio
red cabbage
¼ tsp baking soda (if using radicchio or red cabbage)
dried unsweetened shredded coconut
¼ C powdered sugar
½ tsp milk

liquify

Use one of the following methods create the liquid for your colorful sprinkles:

Fruit Method: Using fresh or frozen fruit, start with one cup of either **raspberries** (red) or **mangoes** (yellow). Use a blender to liquify the fruit into a thick liquid, then pour into a fine strainer to remove any seeds, using a spatula to scrape the bottom occasionally. If using frozen fruit, pour in water, a tablespoon at a time while blending to reach desired consistency. You should get about ½ cup of juice out of the fruit.

Root Vegetable Method: Using **roasted beets** (red), **raw carrots** (yellow), or **spinach** (green), add vegetables to a blender with a dash of water and blend. Continue adding small amounts of water as you blend until the vegetables begin to totally blend and liquify. Then pour the vegetable liquid into a fine strainer or cheesecloth to remove the pulp. You should get about ½ cup of vegetable juice.

Cabbage Method: Chop a small head of either a **radicchio** or **red cabbage** (blue) and add to a medium-size pot on your stovetop and cover with water. Bring to a boil and simmer until the water turns deep purple, about 25 minutes. Remove the radicchio or cabbage, strain the liquid, and add ¼ **teaspoon of baking soda** to the purple liquid. The baking soda turn the liquid from purple to blue!

reduce

Once you have created your rainbow liquids you'll need to reduce them to make them more vibrant. Pour each juice once at a time into a small saucepan and cook over medium heat until it reaches a thick, very vivid paste. This will become your natural food coloring paste.

add+mix

Add **1 tablespoon of shredded coconut** to small bowls (one for each color) and add about a ¼ teaspoon of your natural food coloring paste. Mix thoroughly until the coconut is completely and evenly coated with the color.

spread+dry

Heat a skillet on your stovetop over very low heat and spread the dyed coconut shreds on the skillet to dry the color onto the coconut. Try not to mix the colors when still wet. Cook for about 5 to 8 minutes, watching closely so the coconut doesn't burn. Remove from heat when coconut shavings are dry. You can mix the colored coconut flakes together for a rainbow-sprinkles effect!

whisk+drizzle+sprinkle

Make a sugar glaze. Whisk together ¼ **cup of powdered sugar** and ½ **teaspoon of milk** in a small bowl until smooth. Then spread a small amount of glaze over cooled cupcakes and top with the *Rainbow Glazed Coconut Sprinkles* you just made! The sprinkles will stick to the glaze like glue!

BATTERS: If you're adding ingredients like chocolate chips or fruit to a batter, coat them in a dusting of flour first! This will help the ingredients to stay suspended in the batter and not sink to the bottom.

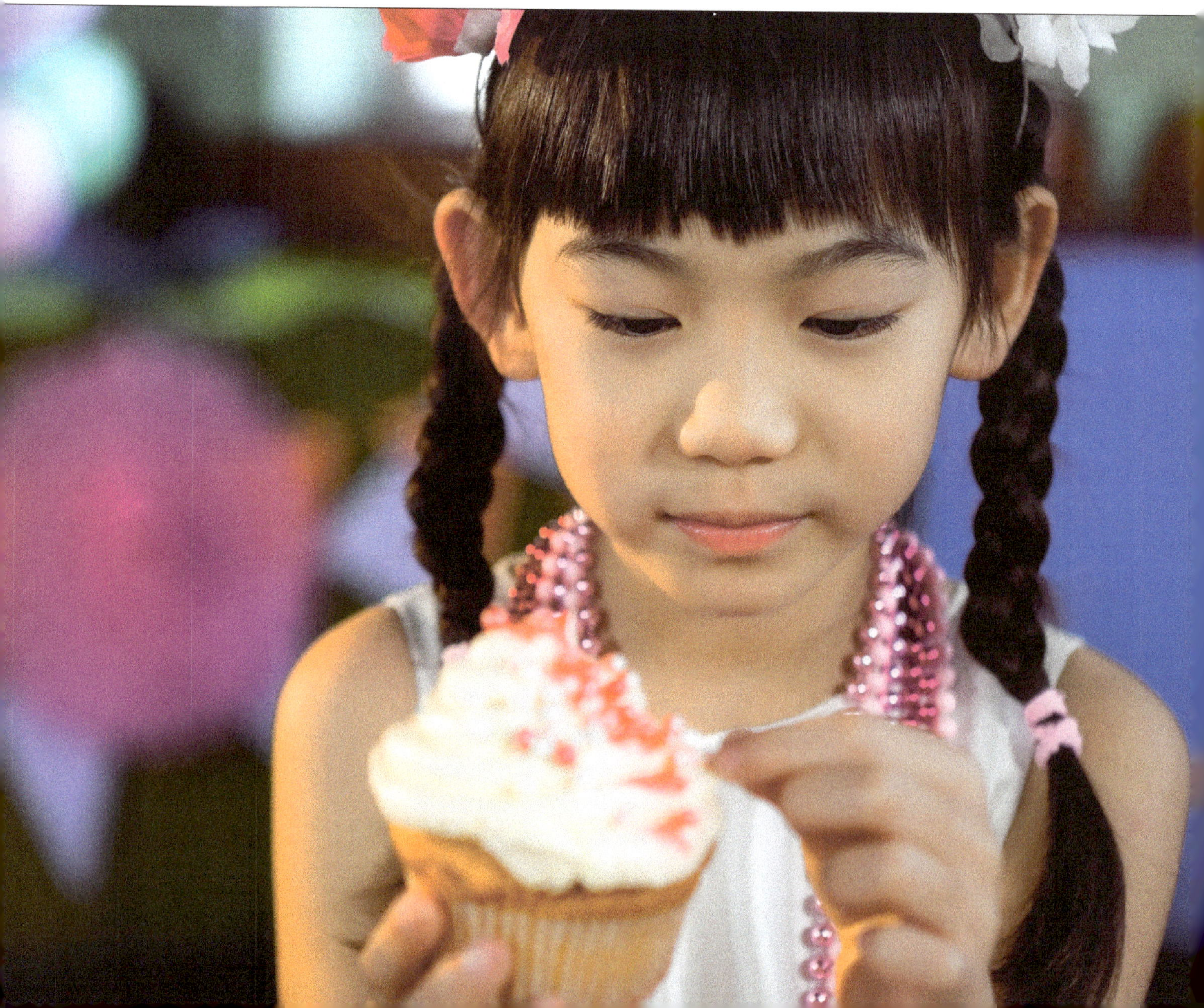

Zany Zucchini Root Beer Cupcakes + Black Pepper Glaze

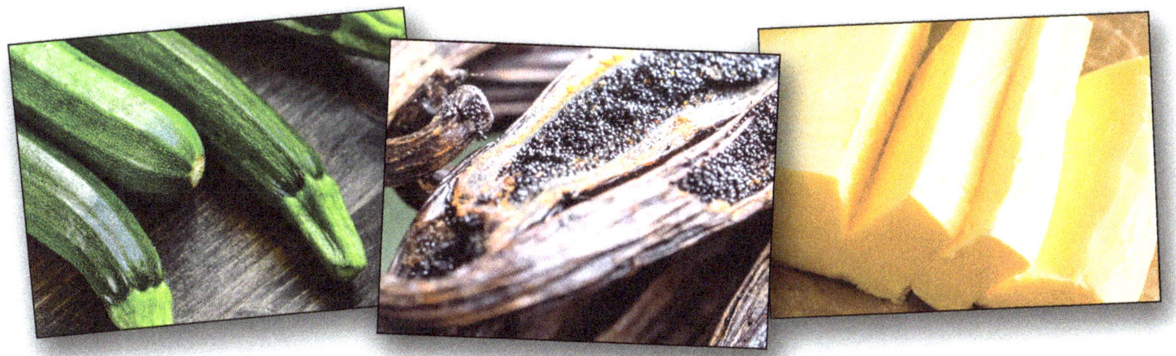

zany zucchini root beer cupcakes

ingredients

1 small zucchini
1¾ C all-purpose flour
1 tsp baking powder
½ tsp baking soda
1 tsp salt
1 C root beer
⅓ C maple syrup/sugar/agave
¼ C unsalted butter
1 T apple cider vinegar
1 tsp vanilla extract

preheat+line

Preheat your oven to 350 degrees F and line a muffin pan with paper liners. Leave your butter out to come to room temperature, or heat in the microwave in 10 to 15 second increments.

grate+squeeze

Grate **1 zucchini** and squeeze out the liquid using a clean dishtowel over the sink. You want to get the extra liquid out of the zucchini so that your cupcakes stay dry and fluffy!

measure+combine

In a large bowl, measure and combine **1¾ cups of flour, 1 teaspoon of baking powder, ½ teaspoon baking of soda,** and **1 teaspoon of salt.** Whisk everything together. Then, in a separate medium bowl, measure and combine **1 cup of root beer, ⅓ cup of maple syrup, ¼ cup of butter** (room temperature), **1 tablespoon of vinegar, 1 teaspoon of vanilla extract,** and ½ **cup of your grated zucchini.** Mix well.

stir+spoon+bake

Stir the wet ingredients into the dry ingredients until just combined, being careful not to over mix. Spoon the batter into your lined muffin pan about ¾ full. Bake in your preheated oven for 15 to 20 minutes, or until a toothpick inserted into the center of a cupcake comes out clean. Very carefully take the cupcakes out of the oven and let cool completely before adding the *Black Pepper Glaze*.

black pepper glaze

ingredients

1 C powdered sugar
1 to 2 T root beer
pinch black pepper

measure+smoosh

To properly smoosh your ingredients, add **1 cup of powdered sugar, 1 to 2 tablespoons of root beer,** and **a pinch of black pepper** to a resealable plastic bag. Seal and smoosh! Continue smooshing until a glaze forms. Add powdered sugar and root beer to your desired consistency.

snip+glaze

Snip the corner of the sealed plastic bag, then squeeze the bag to drizzle the glaze onto the *Zany Zucchini Root Beer Cupcakes* to make fun designs. YUM!

GENERAL BAKING: Oven temperatures can vary greatly, so try using an oven thermometer to accurately measure the inside temperature!

Time for a Laugh!

What did the cupcake say to the fork?

You want a piece of me?

What do you call an island populated by cupcakes?

Desserted!

Hummingbird Cake Pops on a Stick + Fast Pineapple Frosting

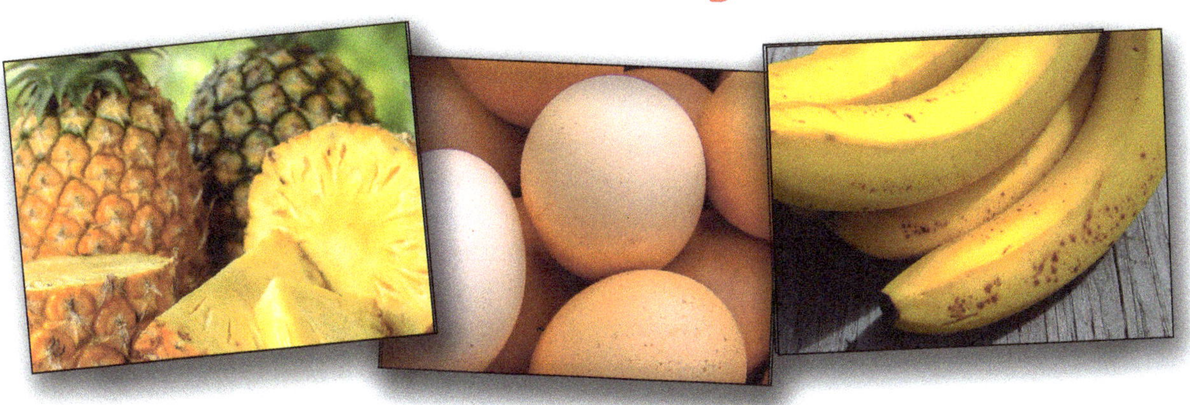

Hummingbird cake is a traditional Jamaican dessert filled with banana, pineapple, and rich spices and topped with a cream cheese frosting. This heavenly cake was named after Jamaica's national bird the Swallow Tail Hummingbird that only lives in this one country!

hummingbird cake pops on a stick

ingredients

- 1½ C all-purpose flour
- ½ C sugar
- ½ C packed brown sugar
- ½ tsp baking soda
- ¼ tsp salt
- ½ tsp cinnamon
- ½ tsp allspice
- ½ C fresh or canned pineapple
- 2 very ripe bananas
- 1 egg
- ½ C vegetable oil (+ more to cook)
- 1 tsp vanilla extract
- popsicle or lollipop sticks

preheat+measure+mix

Preheat your oven to 350 degrees F. Mix the dry ingredients in a large bowl: **1½ cups of flour, ½ cup of sugar, ½ cup of brown sugar, ½ teaspoon of baking soda, ¼ teaspoon of salt, ½ teaspoon of cinnamon**, and **½ teaspoon of allspice.**

chop+mash

Chop ½ **cup of pineapple** and **2 bananas** into tiny pieces and combine in a second large bowl. Mash the chopped fruit with a potato masher.

crack+whisk

Crack **1 egg** in with the mashed fruit, and then add ½ **cup of vegetable oil** and **1 teaspoon of vanilla extract**. Whisk ingredients until well incorporated.

combine+fold

Add the wet ingredients to the dry ingredients bowl and fold until thoroughly blended. With a pastry brush, coat the insides of the wells of your mini-muffin pan with more vegetable oil.

fill+bake

Fill the wells about ¾ full with batter and then bake for 9 to 14 minutes, or until a toothpick inserted in the center of a cake comes out clean. Set aside to cool.

fast and fab pineapple frosting

ingredients

4 oz cream cheese
2 C powdered sugar
1 tsp vanilla extract
1 tsp vegetable oil
pinch salt
1 tsp canned pineapple juice (or 1 T fresh puréed pineapple)

measure+whisk

Soften **4 ounces of cream cheese**. Add cream cheese to **2 cups of powdered sugar, 1 teaspoon of vanilla extract, 1 teaspoon of vegetable oil,** and **a pinch of salt** in a large bowl and whisk together until creamy.

add+incorporate

If using canned pineapple add **1 teaspoon of pineapple juice** from the can into the bowl. If using fresh pineapple, blend **1 tablespoon of puréed pineapple.** Whisk your choice of juice into frosting until smooth and incorporated.

adjust+drizzle

Add more pineapple juice or puréed pineapple as needed to make the frosting your desired consistency. Then drizzle onto your cooled *Hummingbird Cake Pops* and enjoy!

CUPCAKES: Go for a quick scavenger hunt around the house searching for tiny knick-knacks and craft items that you could turn into beautiful, decorative cupcake toppers!

Key Lime Doughnut Holes
+ Lime Syrup Glaze

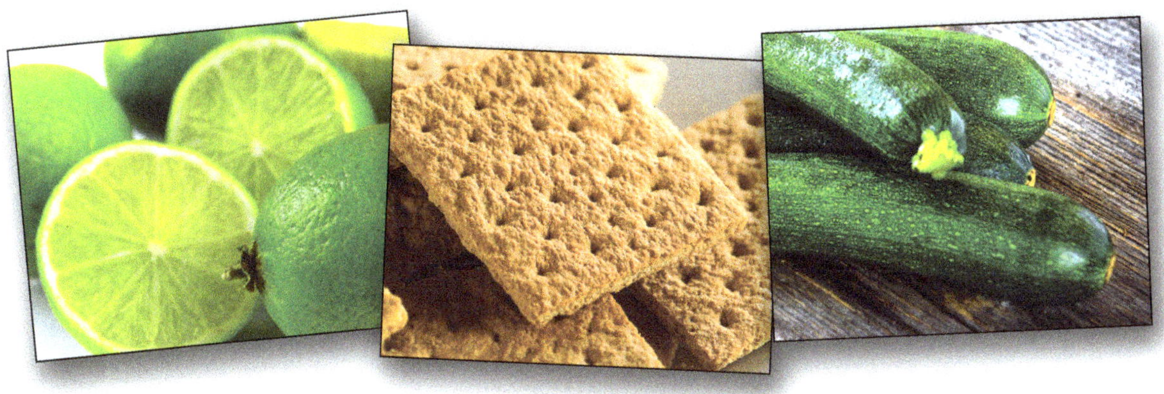

key lime doughnut holes

ingredients

3 T vegetable oil (+ more to cook)
4 to 5 limes (zest and juice)
½ small zucchini
2 to 4 graham crackers
1 C all-purpose flour (+ more if needed)
3 T sugar
2 tsp baking powder
½ tsp salt
1 egg
⅔ C milk (+ more if needed)

preheat+grease

Preheat your oven to 400 degrees F. Pour ¼ **tablespoon of vegetable oil** into the wells of a mini-muffin pan and set aside to be heated later in the oven. This might seem like a lot of oil, but since doughnuts are traditionally deep-fried, this step will allow your doughnut holes to cook evenly on the inside and crisp nicely on the outside when baked.

grate+squeeze

Zest the skin of **1 lime** with a fine grater or zester, avoiding the white part of the lime skin, which can taste bitter. Set zest aside. Lime zest contains oils that are fragrant and full of lime flavor! Squeeze 4 to 5 entire limes to juice them (about ⅔ cups of fresh lime juice) and set to the side. Grate ½ of a zucchini and squeeze out the moisture with a clean dishtowel, discard the liquid. Set aside.

smash+measure

Place **2 to 4 graham crackers** into a sealable plastic bag and smash them into a fine powder with a rolling pin. Set aside. Measure and mix **1 cup of flour, 3 tablespoons of sugar, 2 teaspoons of baking powder,** and ½ **teaspoon of salt** into a big bowl. Next, add ¼ cup of the smashed graham crackers to the flour mixture.

crack+pour

Crack **1 egg** into the flour bowl and mix to combine. Add **⅔ cup of milk** and **3 tablespoons of vegetable oil** to the flour bowl and beat well until smooth. Add the reserved lime zest, lime juice, and zucchini and mix well. If the batter is too thick, add splashes of lime juice or milk and whisk. If the batter is too thin, add 2 tablespoons flour and whisk well.

heat+spoon+bake+turn

When the batter is ready, place the oiled mini muffin pan in the oven until it gets hot. Carefully remove the pan with oven mitts, then spoon 1 tablespoon of the batter into each well. Pop the mini muffin pan back into the oven and bake for 6 to 8 minutes. As soon as the doughnut holes get bubbly and brown around the edges, pull the pan out of the oven and turn the doughnut holes quickly and carefully (a chopstick works great!). Continue baking for 3 to 4 more minutes until doughnuts holes are cooked through. Serve with a drizzle of *Lime Syrup Glaze* and extra crushed graham crackers on top!

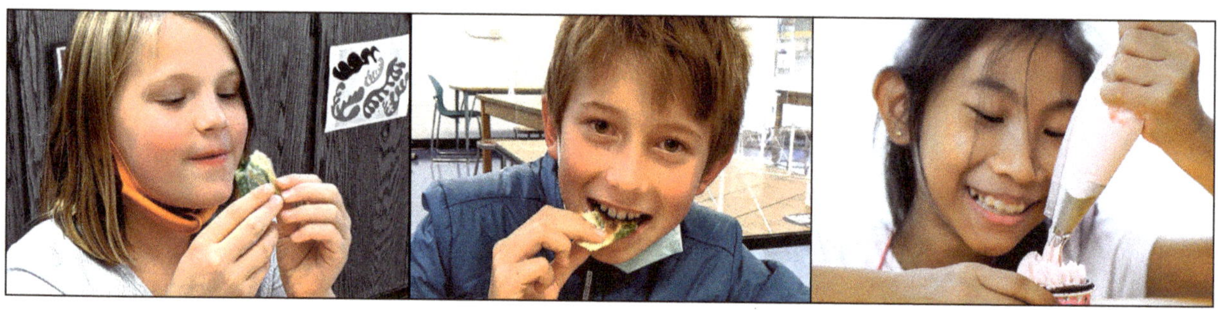

lime syrup glaze

ingredients

½ lime (juice)
½ C powdered sugar
pinch salt

squeeze+pinch+whisk

Squeeze **the juice from** ½ **of a lime** into a bowl. Whisk ½ **cup powdered sugar** and **a pinch of salt** into the lime juice and continue whisking until combined. Whisk in more lime juice or powdered sugar if needed to get the right consistency for drizzling. ENJOY!

Sassy Sweet Potato Brownies + Super Simple Sweet Potato Frosting

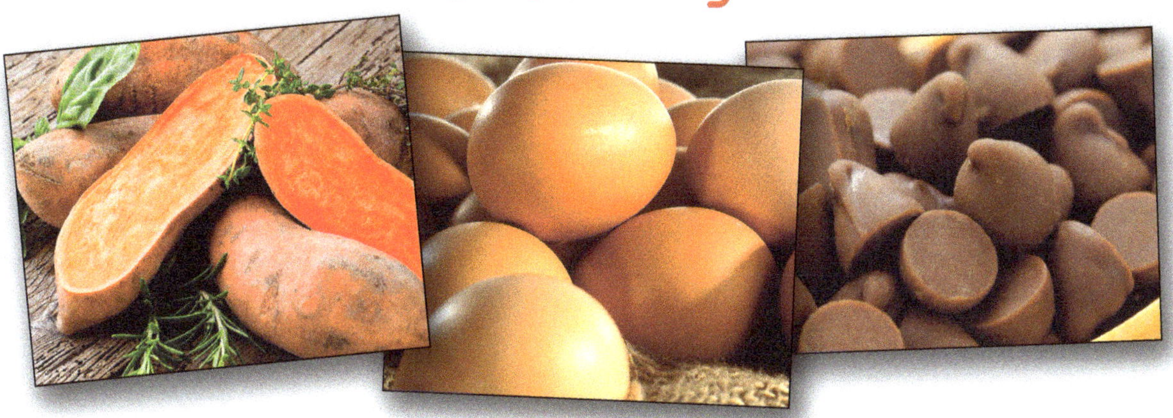

sassy sweet potato brownies

ingredients

2 large sweet potatoes
2 eggs
½ C butter (room temperature)
¾ C sugar
1 tsp vanilla extract
¼ C chocolate chips (+ more for topping)
¼ C unsweetened cocoa powder
¼ C all-purpose flour
1½ tsp baking soda
⅛ tsp salt

cook + cool

Precook **2 sweet potatoes** by either boiling or baking then aside to cool. Set aside butter to become room temperature.

To boil: Chop potatoes into large chunks. Fill a saucepan with enough water to cover the potatoes, bring to a boil, and then add the potatoes. Cover and cook for 10 to 12 minutes or until just tender when pierced with a fork.

To bake: Preheat oven to 400 degrees F. Bake potatoes for 45 minutes, or until the outside of the potatoes have darkened and the insides are soft.

preheat+chop+mash

Preheat your oven to 350 degrees F. Grease an 8x8 pan and set aside. Peel the skin off your cooked sweet potatoes and chop them into chunks. Add 1 cup of sweet potato to a large bowl. Mash with a potato masher until smooth.

add+whisk

Add the rest of the wet ingredients to the large bowl: **2 eggs, ½ cup of butter** (room temperature), ¾ **cup of sugar, 1 teaspoon of vanilla extract,** and ¼ **cup of chocolate chips** and whisk them together.

measure+combine+mix

In another large bowl, measure and combine the dry ingredients: ¼ **cup of cocoa powder,** ¼ **cup of flour, 1½ teaspoons of baking soda,** and ⅛ **teaspoon of salt.** Mix very well, making sure the baking soda is evenly distributed.

add+whisk

Add the dry ingredients to the wet ingredients bowl (not the other way around—this will make for a more delicate brownie!). Whisk ingredients until smooth.

pour+bake

Pour the brownie batter into a greased 8x8 pan and pop them into your preheated oven. Cook for 20 to 25 minutes.

cool+frost

Once brownies are finished baking, remove them from the oven and let sit until cool to the touch. Spread *Super Simple Sweet Potato Frosting* over the brownies and sprinkle with chocolate chips if desired. Cut and sprinkle with a few chocolate chips, if you like, and then cut and enjoy!

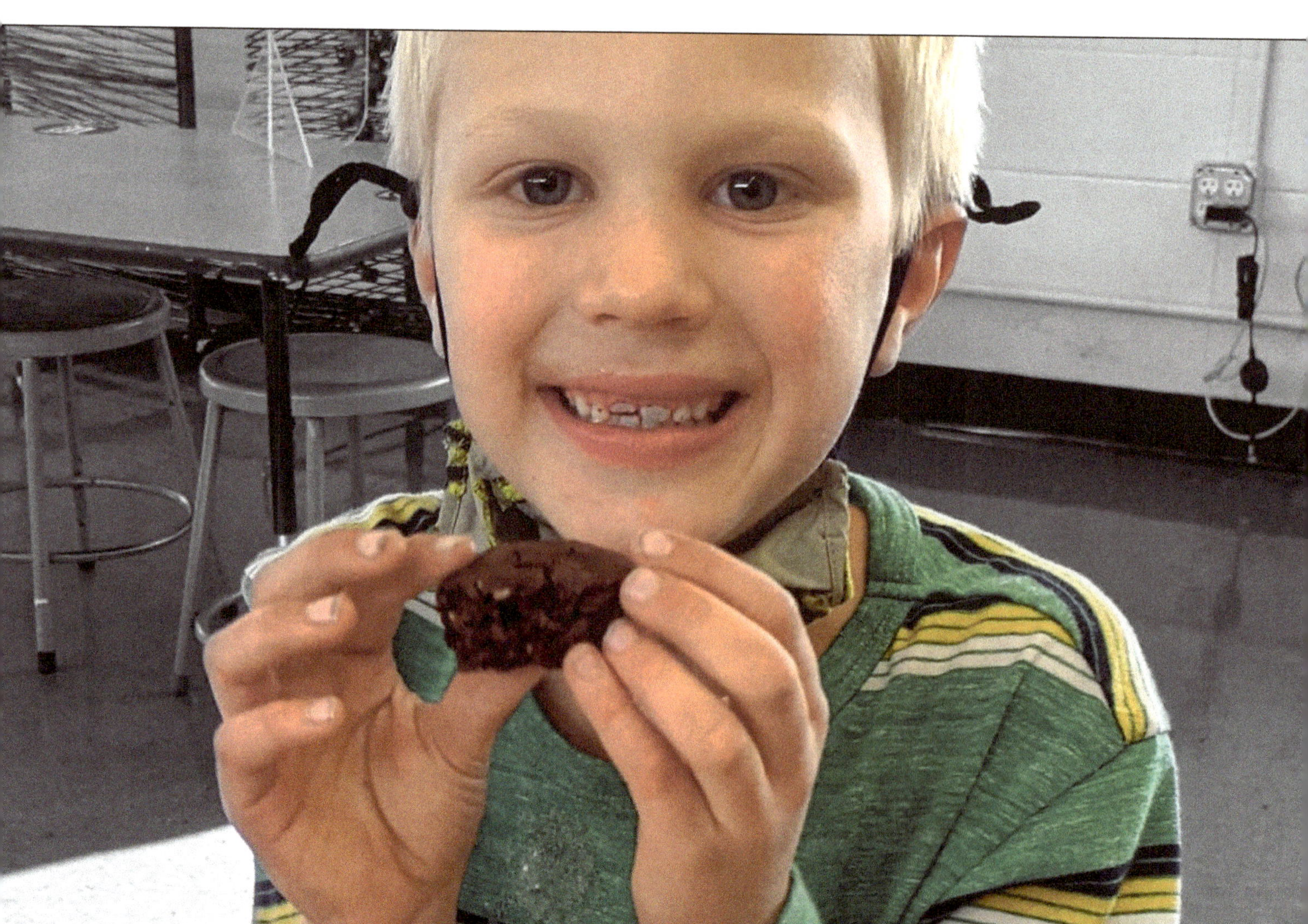

super simple sweet potato frosting

ingredients

2 T unsweetened cocoa powder
1 C powdered sugar
pinch salt
3 T cooked sweet potato
3 T butter
¼ tsp vanilla extract
handful chocolate chips (optional)

measure+combine+whisk

Measure and combine **2 tablespoons of cocoa powder, 1 cup of powdered sugar,** and **a pinch of salt** in a medium bowl and whisk until well combined.

add+blend

Add **3 tablespoons of cooked sweet potato, 3 tablespoons of butter,** and ¼ **teaspoon of vanilla extract** and blend until smooth. If you want even more chocolate, you can sprinkle a **handful of chocolate chips** over the cooled brownies!

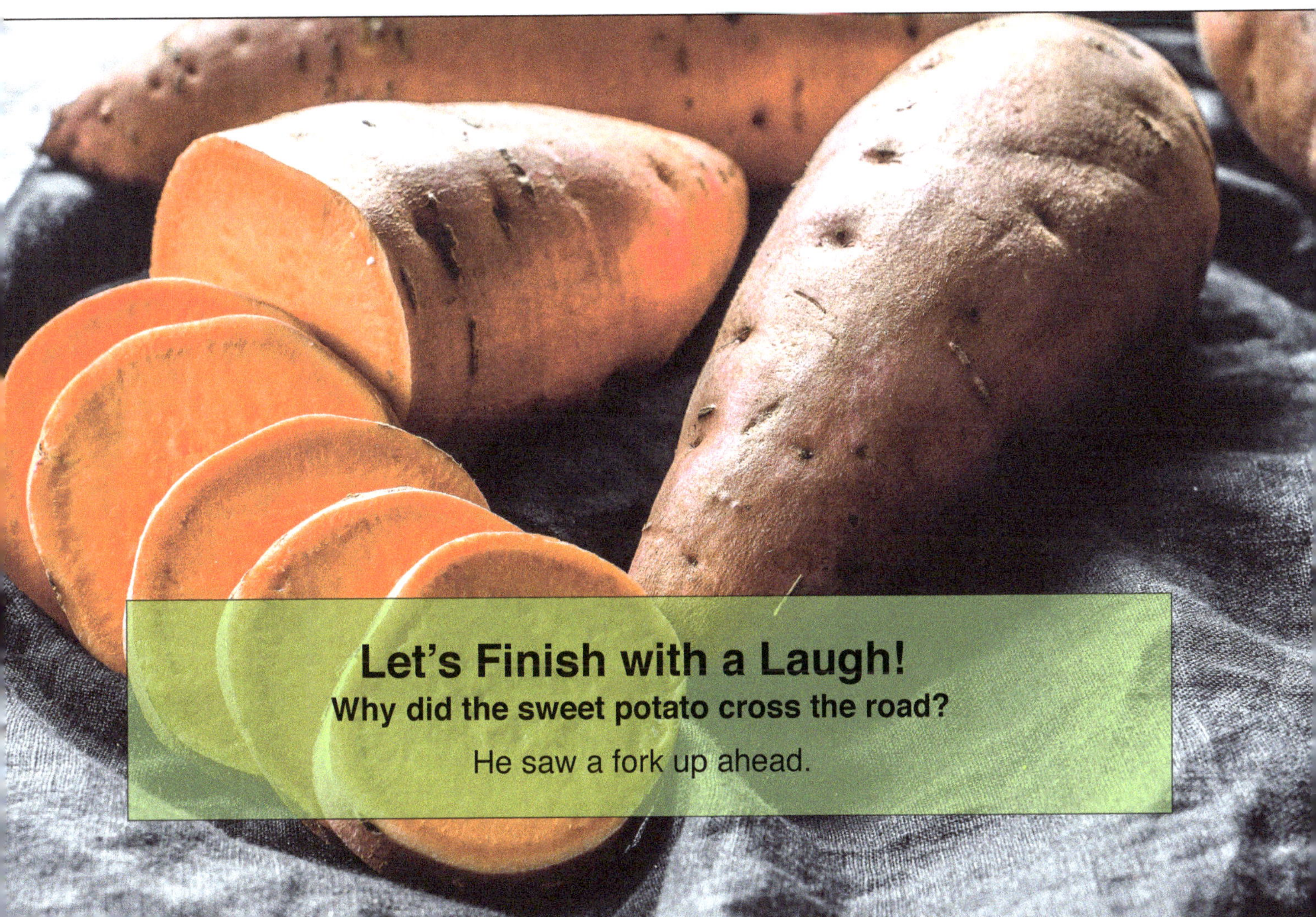

Let's Finish with a Laugh!

Why did the sweet potato cross the road?

He saw a fork up ahead.

Mini Apple Carrot Cinnamon Rolls + Carrot Yogurt Glaze

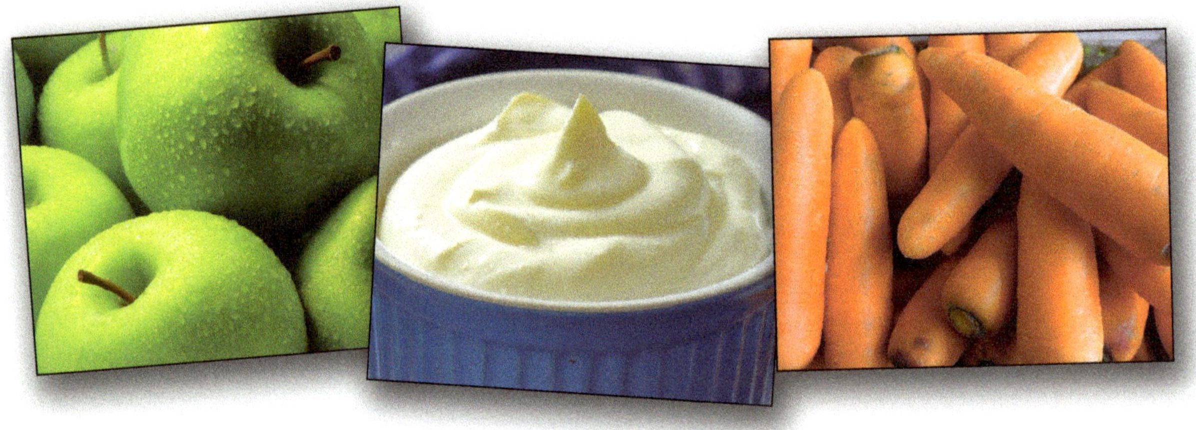

mini apple carrot cinnamon rolls

ingredients

4 T unsalted butter
⅓ + ⅓ C packed brown sugar
3 tsp cinnamon
1 Granny Smith apple
2 C all-purpose flour
4 tsp baking powder
1 tsp sea salt
3 T whole milk Greek yogurt (+ more for dough if needed)
1 large carrot
½ to ¾ C whole milk

preheat+mix+chop

Preheat your oven to 375 degrees F and grease a muffin pan. Soften **4 tablespoons of butter**. To make the filling, have your kids combine, softened butter, **⅓ cup of brown sugar,** and **3 teaspoons of cinnamon** in a small bowl and mix until it forms a crumbly mixture. Cut **1 apple** in half and chop into tiny, tiny pieces and add to the filling. Set aside.

mix+grate+knead

In a large bowl, have kids combine **2 cups of flour, ⅓ cup of brown sugar, 4 teaspoons of baking powder, 1 teaspoon of sea salt,** and **3 tablespoons of yogurt** and mix together with a wooden spoon or clean heads until dough comes together! Add up to 2 tablespoons of extra yogurt if the dough feels too stiff. Grate **1 carrot** and add a handful of the grated carrot and 3 tablespoons of the filling to the dough. Set the rest of the carrot aside. Add ½ **to ¾ cup of milk** and work with your hands to form a large ball of soft dough.

roll+fill+roll+slice

Turn out carrot dough out onto a lightly floured, flat surface or cutting board. Use a rolling pin to flatten and shape the dough into a large rectangle-ish shape about ¼ of an inch thick. Spread the remaining cinnamon filling evenly on the dough. Starting with one of the longer sides, gently roll to form one large log and slice into 12 small rolls. The thinner the rolls, the faster they cook!

bake+cool

Place the mini cinnamon rolls into the wells of your greased muffin pan and bake until golden brown and puffy, about 15 to 20 minutes. Let cool slightly.

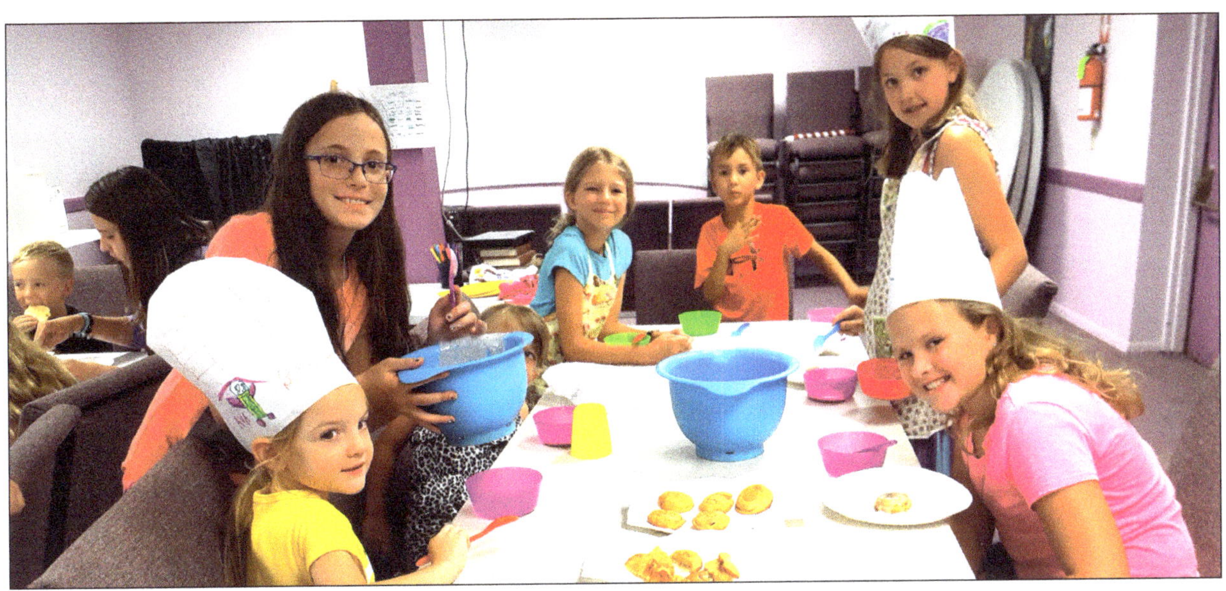

carrot yogurt glaze

ingredients

½ C powdered sugar

¼ C whole milk Greek yogurt

whisk+drizzle

While the cinnamon rolls are baking, make the delicious carrot glaze! In a small mixing bowl, have kids combine ½ **cup of powdered sugar,** ¼ **cup of yogurt**, and 2 tablespoons of the remaining carrots. Whisk until smooth. Drizzle glaze on top of your warm *Mini Apple Carrot Cinnamon Rolls* and ENJOY!

Fabulous Fruity Clafoutis

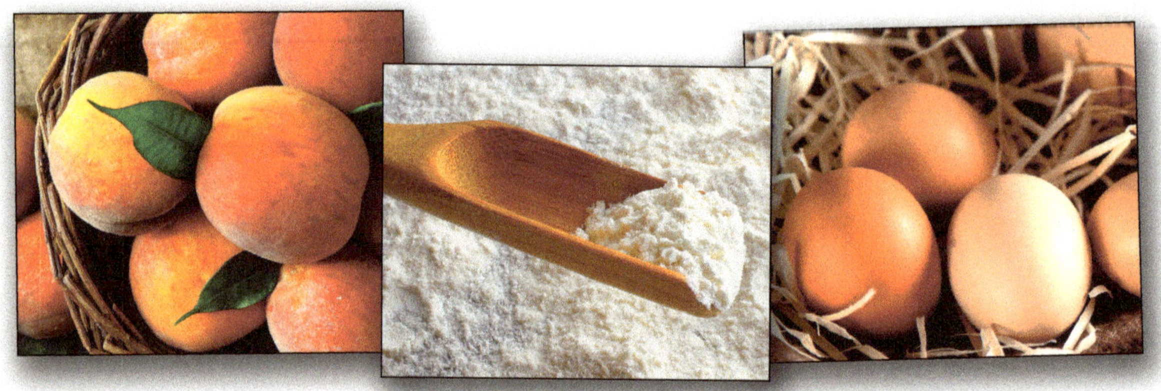

Clafoutis (kla-foo-TEE) is a French dessert made with fruit baked into a creamy-dreamy custard-like batter. It's fancy to say and it's a snap to make! Our favorite fruits for clafoutis are peaches or cherries. You choose what you like best. We always like our Fruity Clafoutis with powdered sugar on top but ice cream, Greek yogurt, or whipped cream are also really delicious!

fabulous fruity clafoutis

ingredients

2 T butter (+ more for greasing skillet)
2 C fruit of your choice
3 eggs
1 C whole milk
¼ + ¼ C white sugar
1 tsp vanilla extract
½ C all-purpose flour
pinch salt
½ lemon (optional)
powdered sugar (optional)

preheat+grease

Preheat your oven to 350 degrees F. Lightly grease a medium-sized, cast-iron skillet or a flameproof baking dish (at least 1½ inches deep) with **butter**.

prep+chop+crack+clean

Wash and dry **2 cups of fruit of your choice** and chop them into small bite-sized pieces, if needed. Set aside. Kids can crack **3 eggs** into a small bowl and set aside. Be sure to wash your hands afterward!

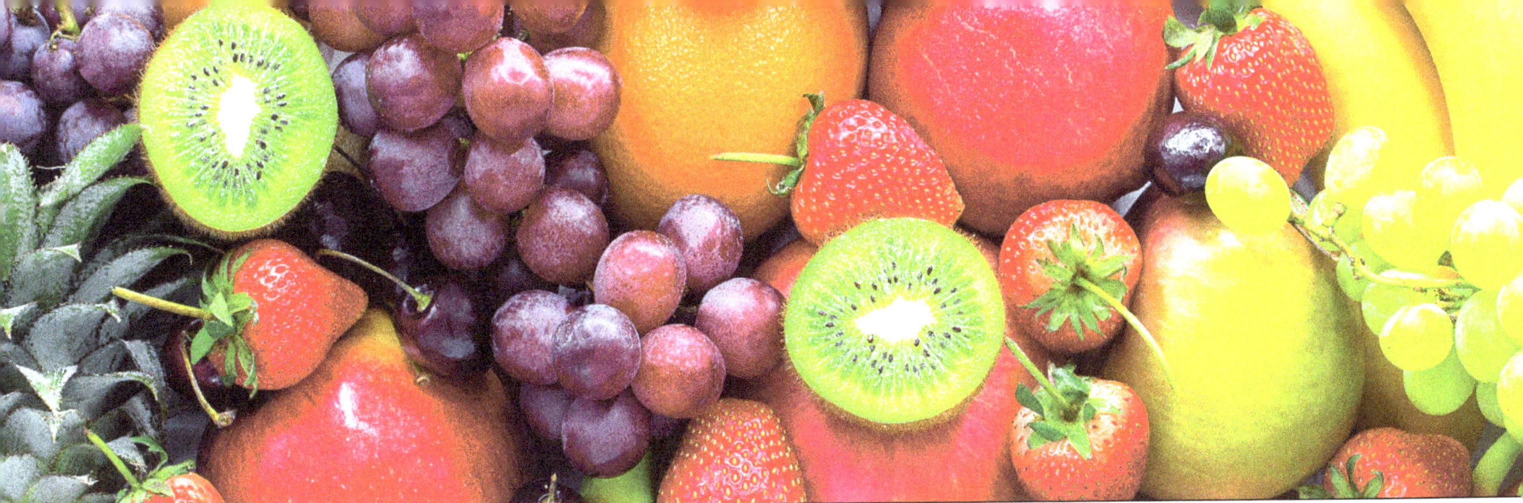

Have fun selecting (at least!) 2 of these fresh and tasty fruits for your clafoutis:

cherries
strawberries
peaches
plums
blackberries
apples
raspberries
blueberries

melt+measure+add

In a microwave-safe bowl or mug, melt 2 tablespoons of butter in 20 second increments. Set aside to cool slightly. In a blender, add **1 cup of milk, ¼ cup of sugar, 1 teaspoon of vanilla extract, ½ cup of flour, a pinch of salt, and the butter and eggs**. For an optional kick of flavor, zest ½ **a lemon** and add the lemon zest to your blender.

blend+pour+sprinkle

Blend at top speed with the lid on for 1 minute until smooth and frothy. Pour your batter into your pre-buttered skillet or baking dish. Have kids evenly scatter your fruit over the batter and sprinkle the remaining ¼ **cup of sugar** over top.

bake+test+cool

Carefully place the skillet in the center of the oven and bake for about 50 minutes or until the top of the clafoutis is puffed and browned. Push a toothpick or wooden chopstick into the center to test if the clafoutis is ready. If it comes out clean, it's done! Let cool slightly. Clafoutis is best served warm, not hot, and it will sink slightly as it cools—that's okay!

sprinkle+enjoy

Using a fine mesh strainer or sieve, sprinkle powdered sugar on top just before serving (or serve with the topping of your choice), dig in, and ENJOY!

Mealtime Chatter: How will you make this recipe next time? Same fruits? A mixture of fruits? Add in some chocolate chips?

Sensational Show Stopping Sugar Cookies + Delightfully Decorative Icings + Best Buttercream Frosting

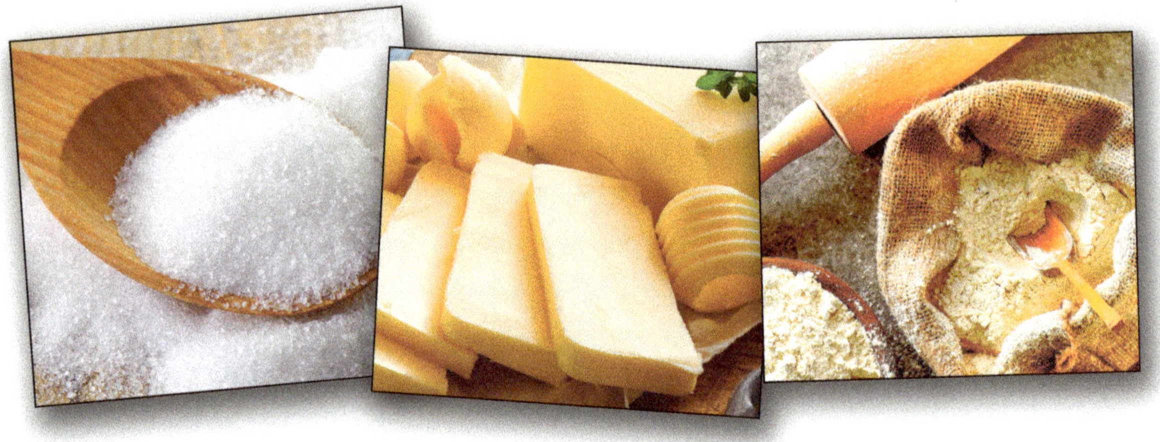

"Cookies are made of butter and love."- Norwegian Proverb.

Sticky Fingers Cooking's Chef Robin and Chef Justin, a mom and son team, shared this special family sugar cookie recipe. It is Robin's Grannie Frances Alexander's original recipe passed down to her beloved mother, Peggy. Chef Robin remembers making these as a child no matter where she moved to, it was something that always connected her to her extended family, even in a new home and in a new city. Now over four generations of Robin's family cherish this recipe and its significant history. That's what baking together can do.

COOKIES: For perfectly baked cookies, take them out of the oven just before the edges brown. The cookies will continue to cook outside the oven, which is called "carry-over cooking."

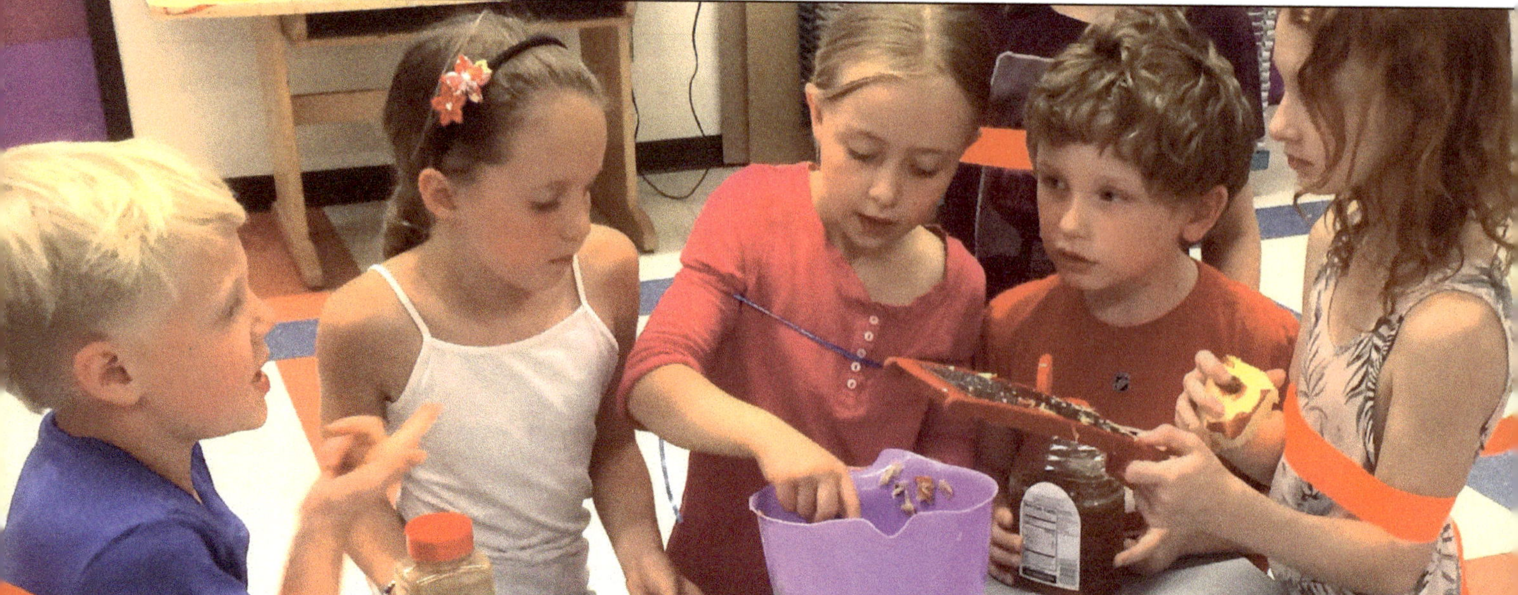

sensational show stopping sugar cookies

ingredients

½ C (1 stick) unsalted butter
¾ C white sugar
1 large egg (sub 1 T ground flaxseed + 3 tsp water for egg-free)
1 T milk (sub soy or rice milk)
1 tsp vanilla extract
2 C all-purpose flour (sub gluten-free flour)
¼ tsp salt
cookie cutters (or mason jar lid/small cup)

preheat+prepare

Preheat your oven to 350 degrees F. Soften ½ **cup of butter** by letting it sit at room temperature for at least an hour or microwave in 15 second increments (it should give a little when squeezed but not be melted).

cream+crack+beat

To prepare your wet ingredients, use a handheld mixer to cream (evenly combine) the butter and **¾ cup of sugar** in a medium-sized mixing bowl. Crack **1 egg** over a small bowl and add to your creamed butter mixture. Pour in **1 tablespoon of milk** and **1 teaspoon of vanilla extract** and beat on low until combined.

sift+combine+mix

In a separate mixing bowl, use a fine mesh strainer or sieve to sift **2 cups of flour** and ¼ **teaspoon of salt** (sifting your dry ingredients makes the dough light and airy!). Carefully pour the dry ingredients into the wet ingredients bit by bit. Mix well with a large spoon or butter spatula at first and continue bringing the dough together with clean hands.

knead+shape+chill

Turn out dough out onto a clean, flat surface and knead (pushing with the palms of your hands) until all the flour disappears and you have a smooth dough. Shape into a big ball, return the dough to the bowl, cover, and chill in the refrigerator for 20 minutes.

roll+cut+bake

Lightly flour a cutting board or countertop. Remove the dough from the refrigerator and begin to flatten the ball with your hands (this will make rolling the dough easier!). Use a rolling pin to roll the dough to ¼ of an inch thick. If the dough starts sticking, add just a bit more flour to your countertop. Use a cookie cutter to punch out your shapes and place on an ungreased baking sheet. Bake 10 to 12 minutes. Remove cookies from the oven, let cool for a minute, and then leave to completely cool on a wire rack until you are ready to decorate!

option 1: ice your cookies! delightfully decorative icings

ingredients

border icing
1 C powdered sugar
2 to 2½ T milk (or water)
½ tsp vanilla extract (or other flavor extract)
food coloring (optional)
piping bags or plastic sandwich bags

flood icing
1 C powdered sugar
2½ to 3 T milk (or water)
½ tsp vanilla extract (or other flavor extract)
food coloring (optional)
piping bags or plastic sandwich bags

measure+stir+color

To ice your sugar cookies, we have two different icings you'll need to prepare. They use the same ingredients but slightly altered measurements because the consistencies will be different.

border icing

To make border icing, add **1 cup of powdered sugar, 2 tablespoons of milk,** and ½ **a teaspoon of vanilla extract** into a small bowl. Stir with a spoon or fork until smooth. Add a couple drops of food coloring, if desired! The icing should be just thick enough to pour but not running (border icing is piped along the edges of cookies to hold thinner flood icing inside).

flood icing

To make your flood icing, add 1 cup of powdered sugar, 2½ to 3 tablespoons of milk, and ½ a teaspoon of vanilla extract into a second small bowl. Stir with a spoon or fork until smooth and add any food coloring, if you want! The icing should drizzle easily when you pick up with spoon or fork. If the icing is still too thick, add more milk, ¼ of a teaspoon at a time, until you reach the desired consistency.

bag+squeeze+repeat

Open two piping bags or plastic sandwich bags and prop them up in a small cup. Use a small rubber spatula or spoon to scoop the border icing out of the bowl and into the first bag. Squeeze the icing down to the corner and twist or fold the bag closed. Repeat this process for the flood icing in the second bag. You'll notice the flood icing will pour much more easily into the bag than the border icing – that's good!

snip+border

Now for the REALLY fun part: decorating! Use scissors to snip the end of the border icing bag. Think about how thin you want your border to be (if the hole is too small, it might be difficult to squeeze the border icing). Using both hands for better control, gently squeeze and pipe the icing around the edges of your cookies (make sure you seal off any holes where flood icing could ooze out!). Let the borders dry slightly before flooding. Repeat with all cookies.

option 2: frost your cookies!
best buttercream frosting

ingredients

1 C (2 sticks) unsalted butter
2 lbs powdered sugar
1 T vanilla extract
¼ to ⅓ C whole milk
food coloring (optional)
piping bag or plastic sandwich bag (optional)
sprinkles (optional)

soften+prepare

Bring **1 cup of butter** to room temperature by letting it sit out for at least an hour or microwaving in 15 second increments. The butter should give a little when squeezed but not be melted. Add to a large mixing bowl.

cream+measure+beat

Half a cup by half a cup, add **2 pounds of powdered sugar** to the bowl and beat with a handheld or stand mixer in between each addition until all the sugar disappears (if you add in all the sugar in at once, you'll have a messy time, and the frosting may seize up!). Pour in **1 tablespoon of vanilla extract** and beat until combined. Slowly add **¼ to ⅓ cup of milk** by the tablespoon until frosting is fluffy and smooth! Add any food coloring at this stage, if desired.

frost+eat

We have two ways for you to decorate your sugar cookies with frosting. You can either pipe them following the same piping process for the border icing, or you can smear and sprinkle. It's up to you, you creative chefs—both ways are beautiful and delicious! To smear, use a butter knife to plop a dollop of frosting onto each cookie. Spread and smooth your frosting this way and that! To finish, add your favorite sprinkles or our tasty *Rainbow Glazed Coconut Sprinkles* on page 17.

Let's Finish with a Laugh!

What do you get when you use a deer-shaped cookie cutter?

Cookie Doe!

"A balanced diet is a cookie in each hand."

- Barbara Johnson

Cheerful Chocolate Chip Celebration Mug Cake

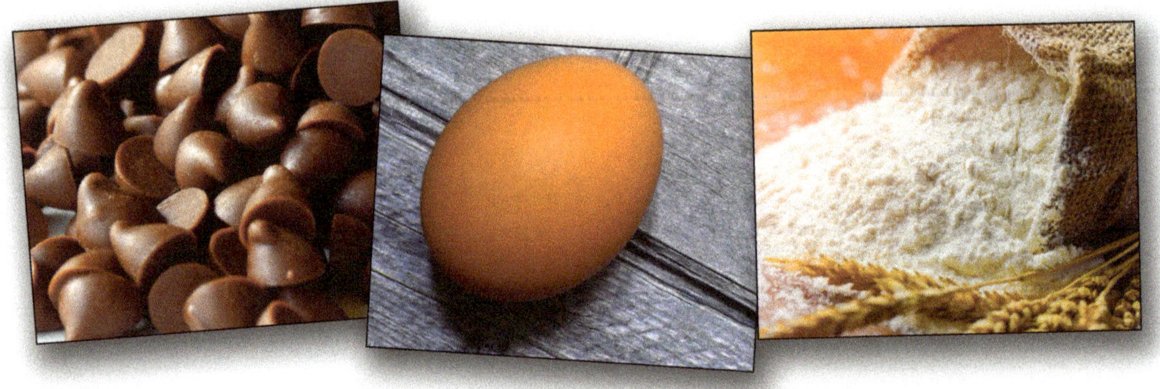

cheerful chocolate chip celebration mug cake

ingredients

1 T unsalted butter
1 T maple syrup
1 tsp brown sugar
½ tsp vanilla extract
pinch salt
1 egg
3 T all-purpose flour
1 T chocolate chips
microwave safe mug

melt+measure

Microwave **1 tablespoon of unsalted butter** in a microwave-safe mug for 30 to 40 seconds until it melts. Use a potholder or towel to carefully remove the mug from the microwave. Add **1 tablespoon of maple syrup, 1 teaspoon of packed brown sugar, a ½ teaspoon of vanilla extract,** and **a pinch of salt.**

crack+separate+mix

Have kids crack **1 egg** over a small bowl and separate the whites from the yolk. Add the yolk to your mug and discard the whites. Mix the ingredients well!

measure+mix+fold+microwave

Mix **3 tablespoons of flour** to your mug mixture until all traces of flour disappear. Fold in **1 heaping tablespoon of chocolate chips**. Cover the mug with a damp paper towel or a dishtowel and microwave on high for 30 seconds. Let rest for 10 seconds. Then microwave for a final 20 seconds. Remove the mug with potholders, let cool slightly, and DIG IN!

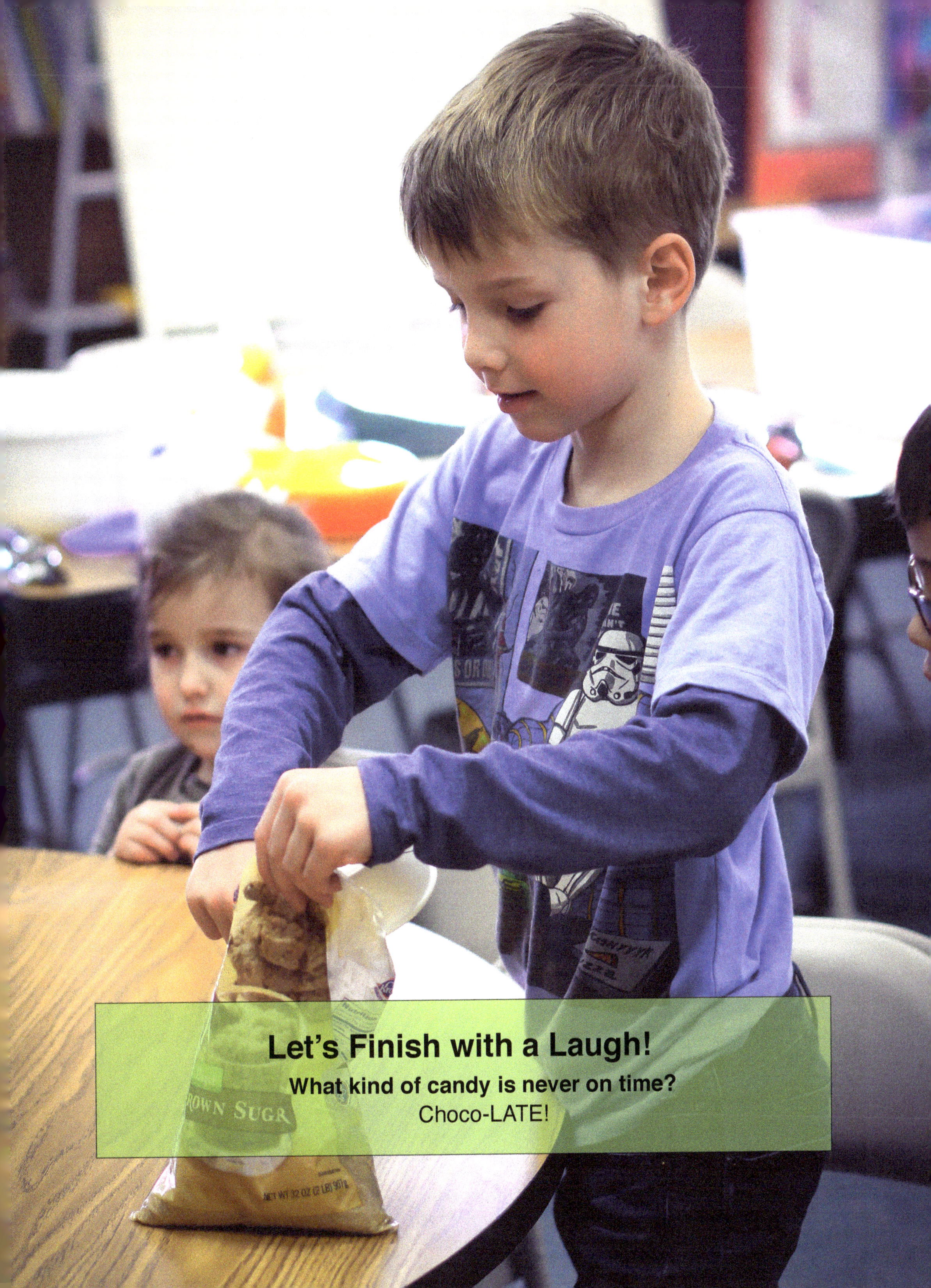

Let's Finish with a Laugh!

What kind of candy is never on time?

Choco-LATE!

Strawberry Banana Birthday Pudding Cake + Sweetly Whipped Strawberry Cream

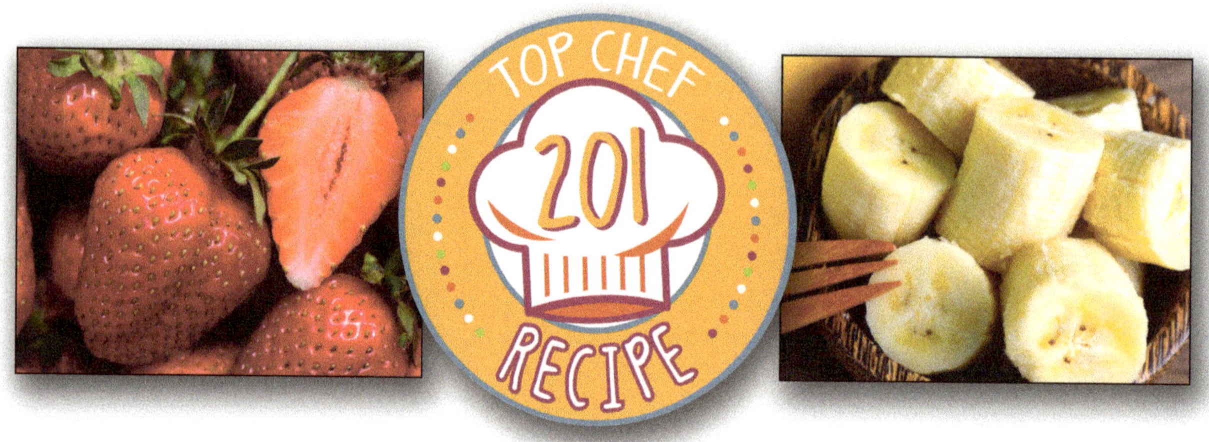

strawberry banana birthday pudding cake

ingredients

1 or 2 ripe strawberries
1½ T butter
microwave-safe mug
2 T packed brown sugar
¼ tsp vanilla extract
2 T full-fat Greek yogurt
1 egg
1 very ripe banana
¼ C all-purpose (or whole wheat flour)
¼ tsp baking powder
pinch salt

BE CAREFUL! Mug cakes are like molten lava straight out of the microwave. Be sure to wait a few minutes to let them cool before eating.

chop+measure+cut

Chop **1 to 2 strawberries** into small pieces and set aside. Measure and cut **1½ tablespoons of butter** from a stick.

WHIPPED CREAM: When shaking whipped cream together, pop your glass or jar into the freezer for a few minutes until cold. Whipped cream doesn't like heat, so shaking in a cold jar will help the whipped cream to stay fluffy!

coat+microwave

Coat the inside of a microwave-safe mug with the **cut butter** and drop the rest of the butter in the bottom of the mug. Microwave for 30 seconds to melt the butter.

measure+crack+whisk

Measure **2 tablespoons of brown sugar, ¼ teaspoon of vanilla extract, and 2 tablespoons of Greek yogurt** to the melted butter. Crack **1 egg** and add to the mug. Whisk to combine everything. Peel **1 banana** and mash it on a plate or in a small bowl with a fork or small whisk. Mash it well! Mix mashed banana and chopped strawberries into your mug.

measure+add+mix

Measure and add ¼ **cup of flour,** ¼ **teaspoon of baking powder,** and **a pinch of salt** to your mug. Mix again!

cover+heat+check

Cover the mug with a damp paper towel and microwave on high for 2 minutes. After 2 minutes, carefully check your mug cake by poking the center with a toothpick. If it doesn't come out clean, microwave for another minute!

sweetly whipped strawberry cream

ingredients

2 ripe strawberries
big pinch sugar
¼ C heavy whipping cream
glass or jar with tight-fitting lid
small pinch salt

chop+sprinkle+mix

Chop **2 strawberries** into tiny pieces. Add to a small bowl, sprinkle a big pinch of sugar over them, and mix to coat the strawberries in sugar. Set aside.

measure+pour+shake

Measure and pour ¼ **cup of whipping cream** to a pint-sized glass or plastic jar and seal with the lid. With one hand over the lid and the other holding the jar, start shaking the jar back and forth, up and down, round and round, and side to side! Your cream will start to thicken after 20 to 30 seconds of shaking. Stop and check the consistency you want your cream to be thick but not as thick as butter.

peel+mash+mix

Add your chopped strawberries, their juices, and a small **pinch of salt** to the jar. Stir to combine. Top your *Strawberry Banana Birthday Pudding Cake* with *Sweetly Whipped Strawberry Cream.*

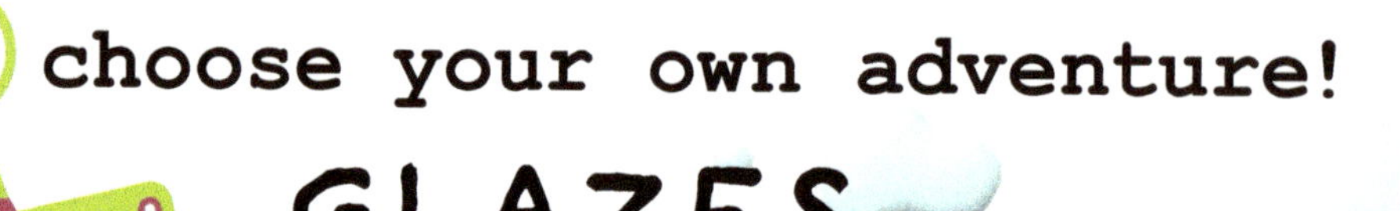

choose your own adventure!

GLAZES + FROSTINGS

glaze + frosting base:

Start with **2 cups of powdered sugar** in a small mixing bowl.

PICK YOUR BASE!

2 tablespoons:

sour cream
softened cream cheese
softened unsalted butter
full fat Greek yogurt

ADD FLAVOR!

teaspoon/s:

vanilla extract
cinnamon
almond extract
coconut extract
mint extract
chocolate sauce

tablespoon/s:

strawberry jam
(or any fruit jam!)
mashed kiwi
mashed peaches
mashed blueberries
pureed pineapple

ADD A LITTLE BIT OF LIQUID! (if needed)
up to 3 tablespoons, depending on consistency:
whole milk
buttermilk
pineapple juice
orange juice
apple juice
MIX IT!
MIX IT REAL GOOD!

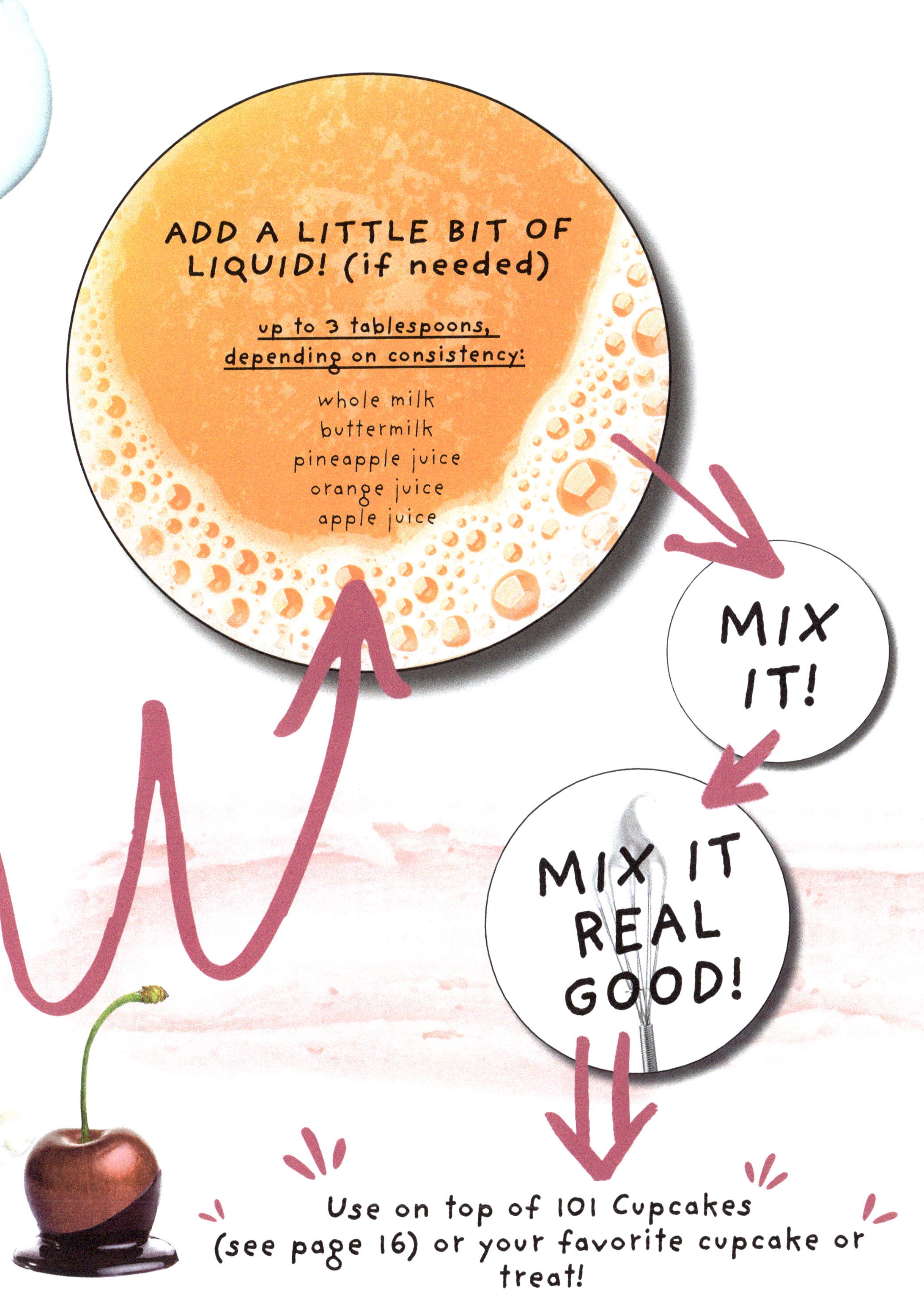

Use on top of 101 Cupcakes (see page 16) or your favorite cupcake or treat!

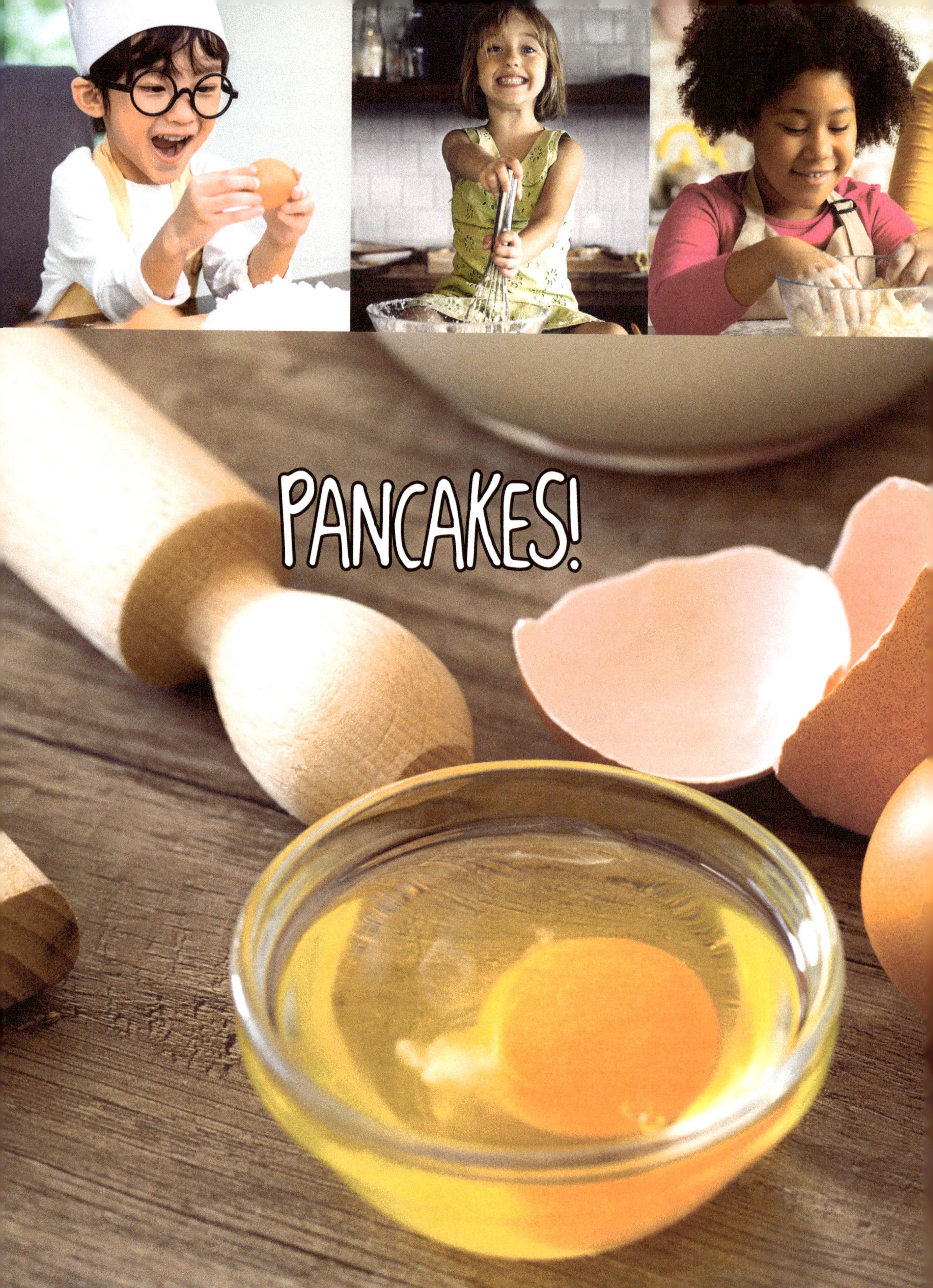
PANCAKES!

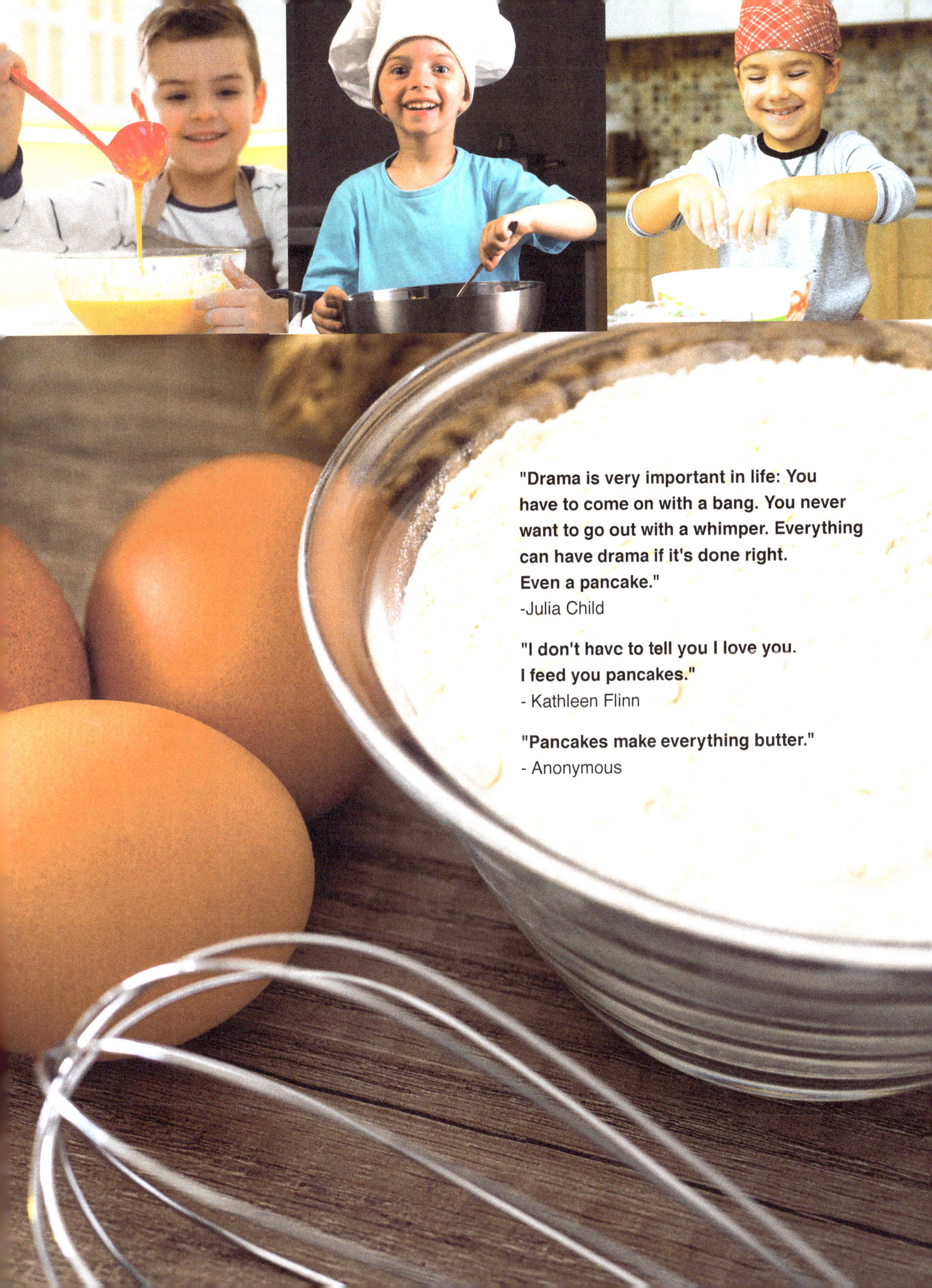

"Drama is very important in life: You have to come on with a bang. You never want to go out with a whimper. Everything can have drama if it's done right. Even a pancake."
-Julia Child

"I don't havc to tell you I love you. I feed you pancakes."
- Kathleen Flinn

"Pancakes make everything butter."
- Anonymous

The Best Flippin' Pancakes Ever (aka Connor Cakes)

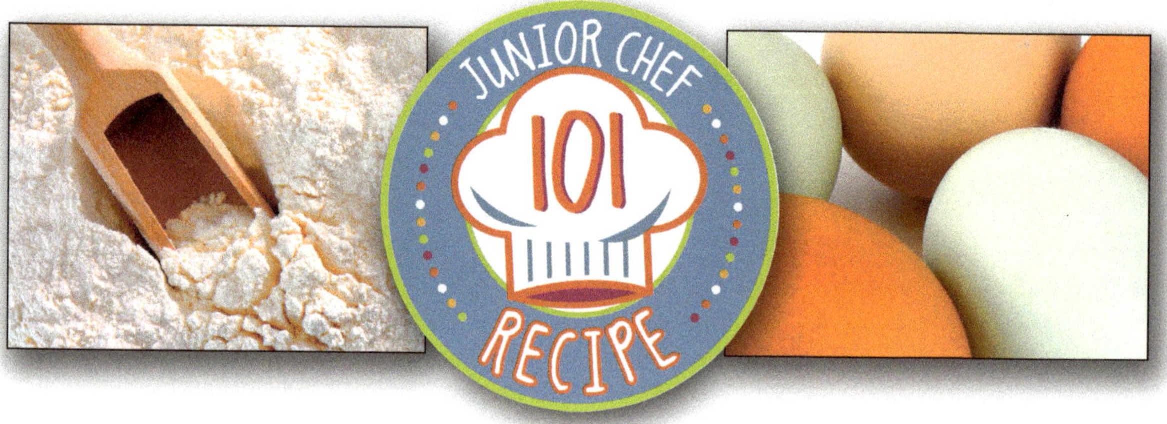

The Connor Cake recipe was shared with me by my dearest friend, Megan. This recipe has been passed down in the Connor Family for generations. Megan remembers her own grandad making these for her on his old plug-in griddle. Megan's dad is now famous amongst his grandkids for making piles of these pancakes whenever he has visitors. Connor Cakes are an always-requested, post- sleepover breakfast requirement at Megan's house. Talk about a pure-pancake-perfection family legacy recipe! They are the best (flipping) pancakes I've ever had.

connor cakes

ingredients

1½ C all-purpose flour
1 tsp baking soda
1 tsp baking powder
2 eggs
2 C buttermilk
½ C vegetable oil

prep+warm

Preheat your oven to 170 F to "warm" and place an oven-safe plate inside to warm up.

measure+whisk

Find a medium-sized bowl and have kids measure and whisk together the **1½ cups of flour, 1**

tsp of baking soda, 1 tsp of baking powder, and **1 tsp of table salt**. Set to the side. This is the dry bowl.

crack+beat

In a smaller bowl, have kids crack and beat **2 eggs** until smooth. Kids should clean their clappers afterward (wash their hands)!

pour+whisk

Have kids pour in the **2 cups of buttermilk** and **½ cup of vegetable oil** in the same bowl with the beaten eggs. You can use the same whisk you used for the dry ingredients. Whisk until smooth. This is the wet bowl.

combine+stir

Kids can pour and mix in the dry bowl mixture directly into the wet bowl in small increments. Gently stir everything together until just combined. Be careful not to overmix your pancake batter!

nap+thicken=fluffy

The batter needs to nap (or rest) for about 10 minutes which is essential because the batter will thicken up when the flour absorbs the liquid, and the baking powder has time to activate with the buttermilk. Thick batter = fluffy pancakes!

bubble+flip+repeat

When bubbles start forming around the edge and at the top of the pancake, flip and cook the other side until puffy, lightly browned, and cooked through (about 2 to 3 minutes). The first pancake is always a test to make sure your stove heat is just right. If your pancake is really dark brown on the outside, turn down your stove. If your pancake is raw in the center and takes longer than 3 to 5 minutes to cook, turn up the heat slightly. After each pancake is cooked, place it in your warm oven on the plate or platter to keep warm before serving. *This step is for adults or master chef kids only!*

serve+customize

To serve, have each person top their pancakes with their favorite toppings! Please see our Un-Recipes on pages 40-41, 86-87, 110-111, 112-113, 130-131 for all the topping inspiration your family needs!

How will you make this recipe next time? Add sliced bananas or berries to the batter? Add in some cinnamon or some chocolate chips?

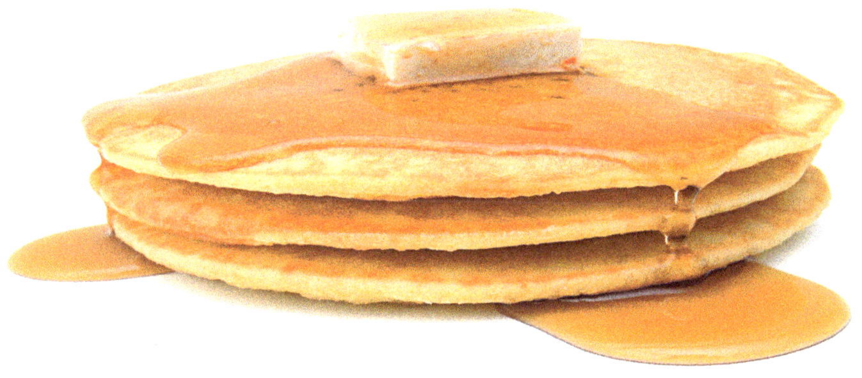

Superhero Crepes

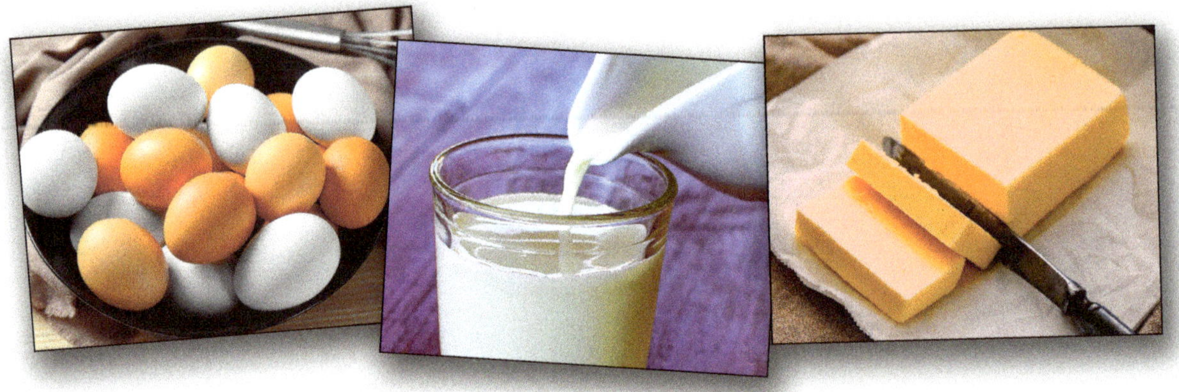

My awesome family member, Paul Noronha, taught me how to make crepes when I was 12 years old in his kitchen in Laguna Niguel, California. Paul has the most amazing stories because he grew up all over the world. Paul taught me the crepe recipe he learned from when he was a teenager in Vienna, Austria. I never forgot the recipe and I credit Paul for adding to my life-long love of cooking! I have adapted Paul's original recipe into the Superhero Crepes to make them as foolproof, fun, and flexible as any Superhero CAPES out there. They'll be sure to save the day for any breakfast, brunch, lunch, snack, dinner, or dessert. Also, your friends and family are bound to call you a Superhero Chef once they taste these crepes that you made for them. Enjoy!

superhero crepes

ingredients

5 large eggs
1 C all-purpose flour
1¾ C milk
¼ C butter
pinch salt

wet+warm

Preheat your oven to "warm" or 170 degrees F and place an oven-safe plate or platter on the middle rack to warm. Wet a clean dish towel and add it to the top of your plate or platter. Melt ¼ **cup of butter**.

crack+beat+clean

Kids can crack and beat **5 eggs** into a large bowl. Beat those eggs up until they are smooth. Kids, be sure to clean your clappers afterward (wash your hands)!

measure+whisk+nap

Kids can measure and add **1 cup of flour, 1¾ cup of milk, ¼ cup of melted butter, and a pinch of salt** into the large bowl, with the eggs, and whisk. This is your crepe batter. Have the batter rest (or nap) for at least 30 minutes and up 48 hours, covered, in the refrigerator. The longer the batter rests, the more elastic, pliable, and forgiving the batter becomes. The flour needs to have time to absorb the eggs and milk. It will be easier to make the crepes (and they'll taste better) after the batter takes a long resting nap.

swirl+flip+feed-the-dog

Crepe time! Heat a nonstick pan, over medium heat. Add a half of a ladleful of batter, just enough to thinly coat the bottom of the pan. Carefully and quickly swirl the batter to evenly coat the bottom and a bit of the side of the pan.

Cook the crepe until the edges begin to brown slightly and pull away from the side of the pan, probably about 30 seconds or so. Flip — this is not as delicate of a process as it seems it should be—So don't worry—cook the crepe about 10 seconds on the other side. This takes a little practice! French people have a saying about crepes, *"le premier crepe est pour le chien"* which says "the first crepe is for the dog" so don't feel bad if you mess the first (or second) crepe up. Turn the heat up or down to make the perfect crepe if it doesn't happen the first or second time you try. This step is for adults or masterchef kids only.

stack+cover

Cook as many crepes as you and your family can eat. Stack crepes on the plate or platter in your warmed oven and cover them, each time, with a wet cloth dish towel until you and your friends and family are ready to eat. Remember that you can save the unused batter in the refrigerator for up to 2 days.

fill+fold+roll+stack

Serve the crepes warm with a whole array of optional fillings and toppings you might like to put in them. Please see our un-recipes on pages 60-61 and 112-113 for filling and topping inspiration! You can fold the crepes in fourths, roll them, or stack them. Remember, crepes can be served sweet (like Nutella and bananas or yogurt and berries) or savory (like: Ham and cheese or tomatoes and basil)

NOTE: Leftover crepes can be layered with wax paper and placed in a plastic bag and stored in the refrigerator for 3 or 4 days. Reheat them in the microwave or in a dry warm skillet, for a quick breakfast or snack. These crepes also freeze really well if stacked between wax paper!

Mealtime Chatter: How will you make this recipe next time? Add sliced bananas or berries to the batter? Add in some cinnamon or some chocolate chips? How will you make this recipe next time? Same fillings? A stack? Rolled? Have you heard about gâteau de crêpe or mille crêpe cakes?

Choose-Your-Own-Adventure Baked Buttermilk Slab Pancakes

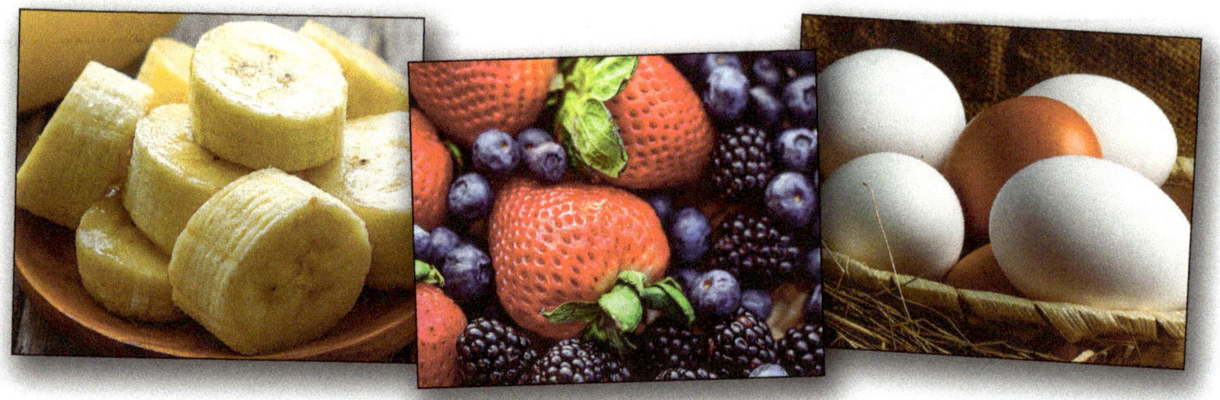

choose-your-own-adventure baked buttermilk slab pancakes

ingredients

butter or olive oil (for cooking)
2½ C whole milk
1 lemon (juice)
½ C unsalted butter
3 C all-purpose flour
2 T baking powder
½ tsp salt
2 eggs
3 T sugar

preheat+measure+mix+melt

Preheat your oven to 425 degrees F. Grease (1) 18x13" sheet pan or (2) 9x13" sheet pans with **butter or olive oil**. Add **2½ cups of milk** and the juice of **1 lemon** to a small bowl, whisk together and set aside. Melt ½ **cup of butter** in the microwave or on the stovetop, and set aside.

measure+whisk+combine

Whisk the following dry ingredients in a medium bowl: **3 cups of flour, 2 tablespoons of baking powder,** and ½ **teaspoon of salt.** In another medium bowl, whisk together **2 eggs**, **3 tablespoons of sugar, melted butter,** and the milk/lemon mixture. Add the dry ingredients to the wet ingredients and mix to combine!

Have fun selecting (at least!) 3 of these fresh and tasty additions to your pancakes:

- dried fruit
- ripe banana
- shredded coconut
- fresh or canned pineapple
- ground cinnamon and sugar
- sliced apple or pear
- orange zest
- chocolate chips
- berries
- pumpkin pie spice

grease+decorate+bake

Pour pancake batter into the pan(s) and spread it out evenly with a spatula.

Now for the fun part: kid chefs can add their chosen pancake **add-in ingredients**! To make a mosaic, decorate in halves or quarters with a different flavor, color, etc. Bake in a preheated oven for 15 minutes or until the pancake is set in the middle and golden brown. YUM!

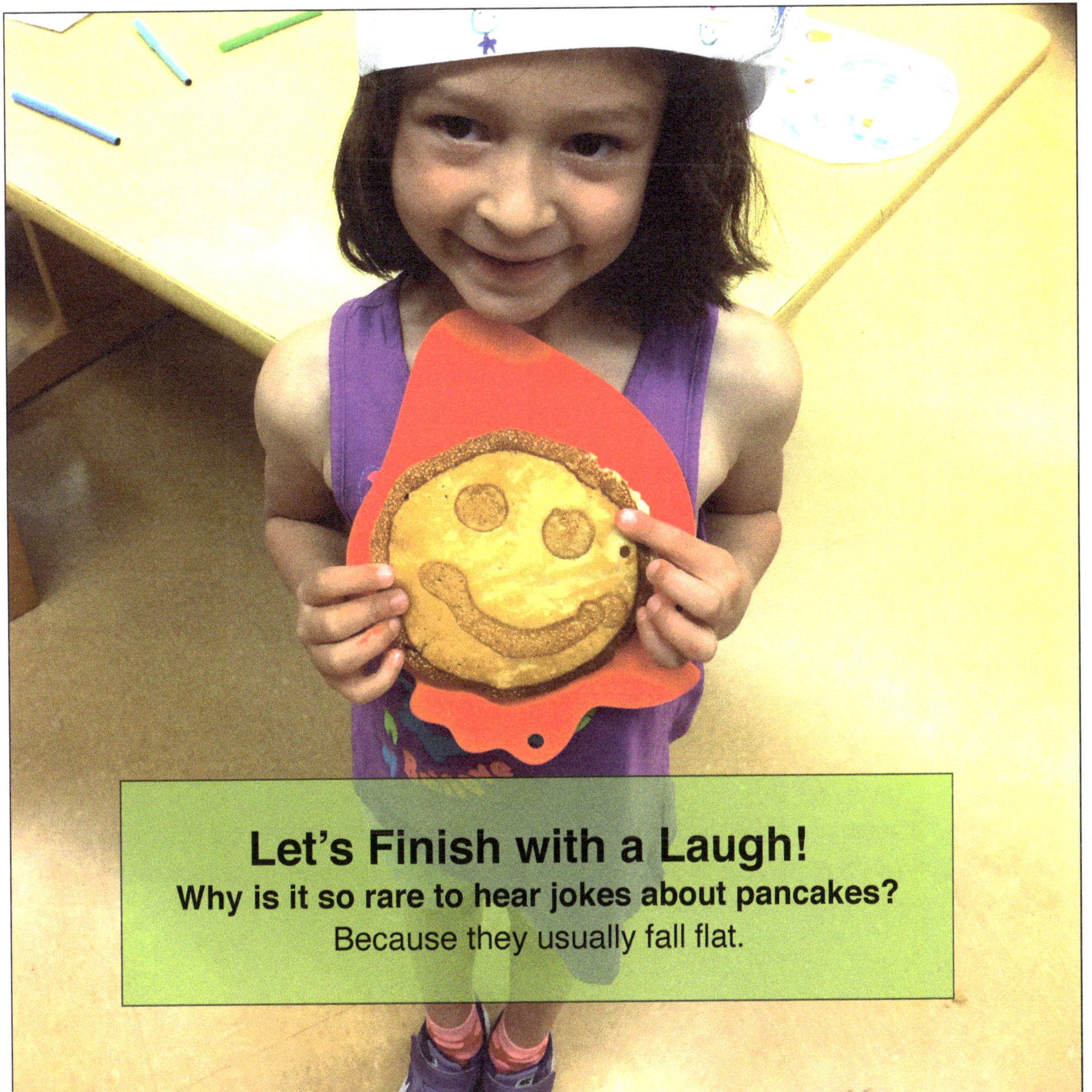

Let's Finish with a Laugh!

Why is it so rare to hear jokes about pancakes?

Because they usually fall flat.

German Black Forest Pancakes + Cherry Glaze

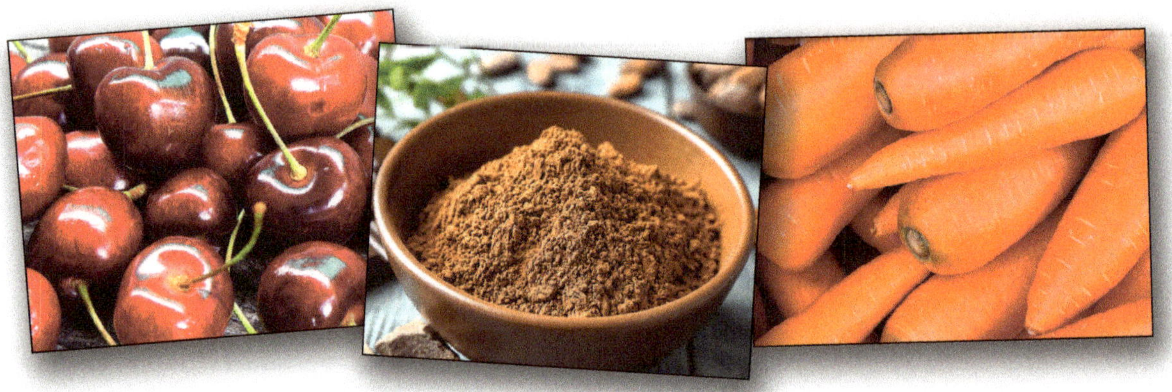

Known in Germany as *Schwarzwälder Kirschtorte* (SHVARTS-vald-er KEERSH-tortuh), this cake is named after the densely wooded Black Forest in southwest Germany known for its cuckoo clocks, dark chocolate, and—you guessed it—cherries!

german black forest pancakes

ingredients

1 C fresh or frozen (thawed) cherries (pitted)
1 carrot
1¼ C all-purpose flour
½ C cocoa powder
1 tsp baking powder
¼ tsp baking soda
½ tsp salt
1 egg
¾ C buttermilk
¼ tsp vanilla extract
3 T unsalted butter
½ C brown sugar
oil (for cooking)

chop+grate

Have your kids chop up **1 cup of cherries** and then grate **1 carrot.** Set aside. Take butter and eggs out of the fridge to get to room temperature.

measure+mix

Measure and mix the dry ingredients in a large bowl: **1¼ cups of flour, ½ cup of cocoa powder, 1 teaspoon of baking powder, ¼ teaspoon of baking soda, ¼ teaspoon of salt.**

crack+combine

Crack and beat **1 egg** into a new large bowl (this will be your wet ingredients bowl). Add **¾ cup of buttermilk, ¼ teaspoon of vanilla extract, 3 tablespoons of butter,** and **½ cup brown sugar** and mix to combine.

whisk+stir

Have your kids whisk the wet ingredients together until light and fluffy, about 3 to 5 minutes. Then, whisk the dry ingredients in with the wet ingredients. Stir in the chopped cherries and the grated carrots.

oil+bubble+flip

Oil a skillet on your stovetop and warm over medium-high heat. Once hot, spoon batter onto the skillet, about 2 tablespoons for each pancake, and wait for bubbles to form. Then flip and cook for another 30 to 60 seconds until cooked on both sides.

cherry glaze

ingredients

handful fresh or frozen (thawed) cherries (pitted + juiced)

1 C powdered sugar

measure+drop+drizzle

Into a new, smaller bowl gradually add **½ to 2 teaspoons of cherry juice** to **1 cup of powdered sugar,** whisking until you get the desired consistency. Drizzle over pancakes and enjoy! As they say "this tastes good" in German, *Es schmeckt* (ehs SHMEH-kt)!

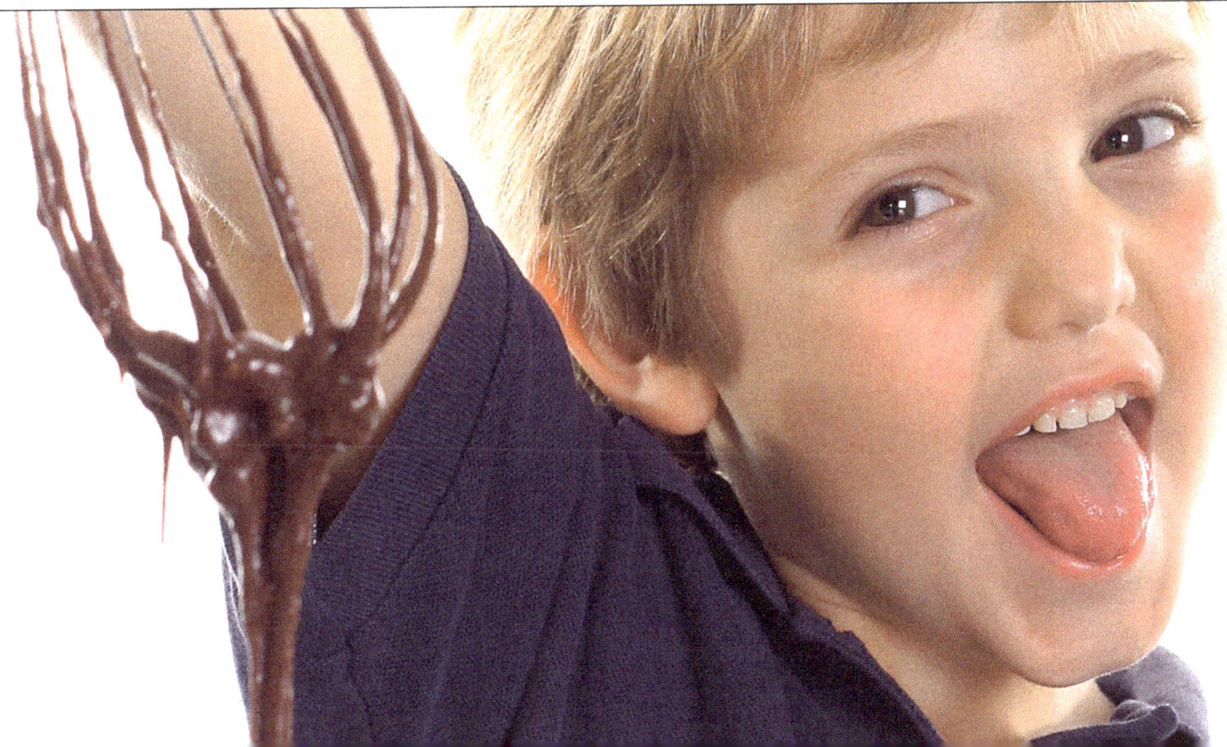

Mini Macaroon Lemon Pancakes

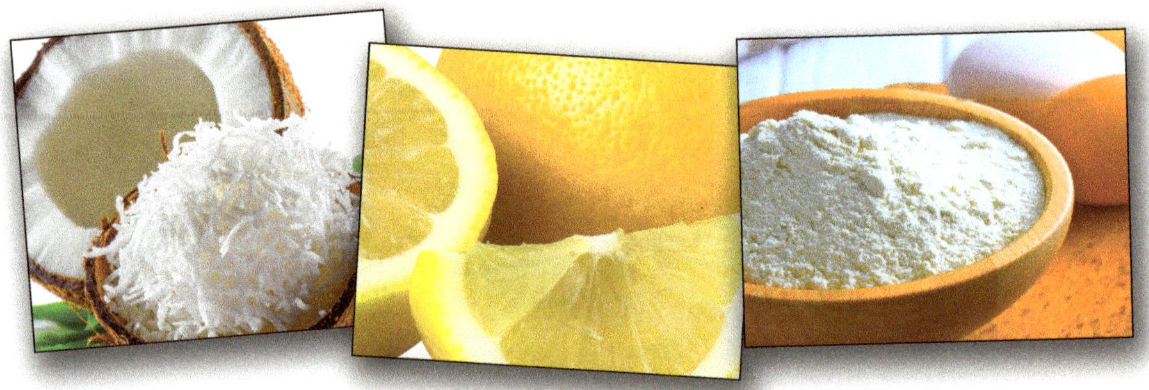

When you see the word macaroon, do you think of those sweet, chewy coconut cookies with a golden crust or those airy, meringue sandwich cookies with buttercream in the middle? It's easy to confuse the two because they are so similar! A macaron is a delicate French sandwich cookie made with egg whites, sugar, almonds, and often coconut while a macaroon is made with many of the same ingredients but comes together differently. When you think of Macarroons, think: homemade, chewy, goldeny, coconutty goodness! That is the inspiration behind these luscious lemon pancakes.

mini macaroon lemon pancakes

ingredients

¼ C dried shredded coconut
1¼ C all-purpose flour (sub gluten-free flour blend)
2 T sugar
1 tsp baking powder
½ tsp baking soda
¼ tsp salt
1 lemon (juice)
1 C coconut milk
1 egg
1 T unsalted butter (sub coconut or vegetable oil) (+ more for cooking)
drizzle honey/maple syrup/agave (optional)

toast+stir

Add ¼ **cup of coconut** to a preheated skillet on your stovetop. Toast for 3 to 5 minutes, stirring a few times with a wooden spoon to ensure an even, light golden color. Turn off heat and remove coconut from skillet when just slightly toasted, being careful not to overcook the coconut and burn it. Add to a large bowl and set aside.

measure+add

Measure and add all of your dry ingredients to the bowl with the toasted coconut: **1¼ cups of flour, 2 tablespoons of sugar, 1 teaspoon of baking powder, ½ teaspoon of baking soda,** and ¼ **teaspoon of salt.** Whisk to combine.

slice+squeeze+curdle

Slice **1 lemon** and squeeze out about 3 tablespoons of juice and add to a large bowl. Add **1 cup of coconut milk** and set aside for a few minutes. It will curdle, but that is what you want! This will be your "buttermilk."

crack+whisk+pour

Crack **1 egg** into the wet bowl and soften **1 tablespoon of butter** (or you could use **coconut oil or vegetable oil**). Whisk well and then pour the wet ingredients into the dry ingredients.

blend+preheat+coat

To make the **toasted coconut pieces** smaller and help them incorporate into the batter, blend the batter for 10 to 20 seconds using an immersion blender, or in a regular blender. Preheat a skillet on your stovetop, adding a pat of butter or some oil to coat the bottom of the pan.

drop+cook+flip

Drop about 2 tablespoons of batter for each pancake onto your hot skillet. Let the pancakes cook until bubbles begin to pop in the center of each pancake, about 2 minutes. Flip the pancakes and cook for an additional minute or so until golden brown. Serve with a **drizzle of honey/maple syrup/agave** on top!

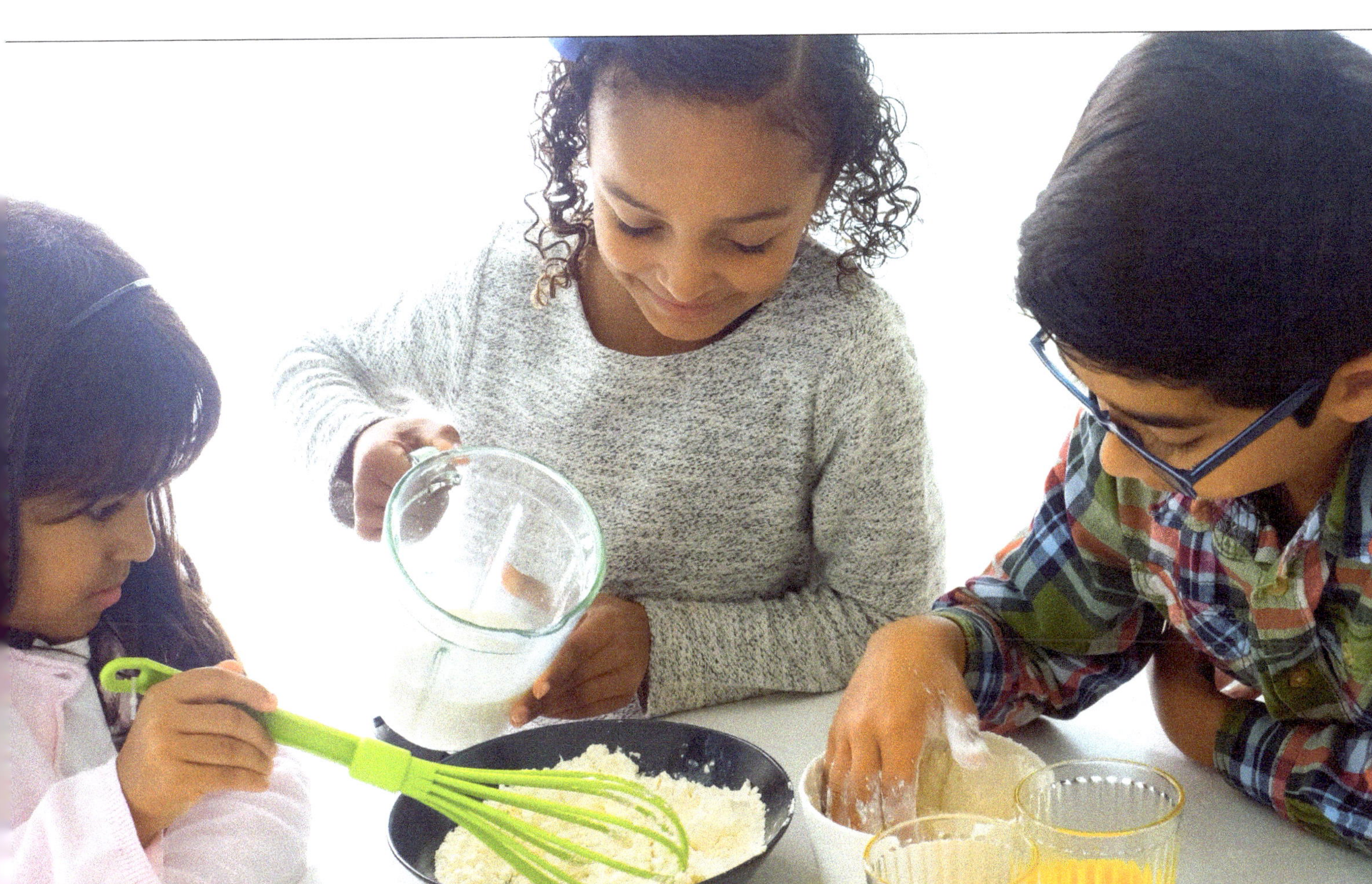

No Sugar Carrot Cake Pancakes + Spiced Cream Cheese Kid-Made Butter

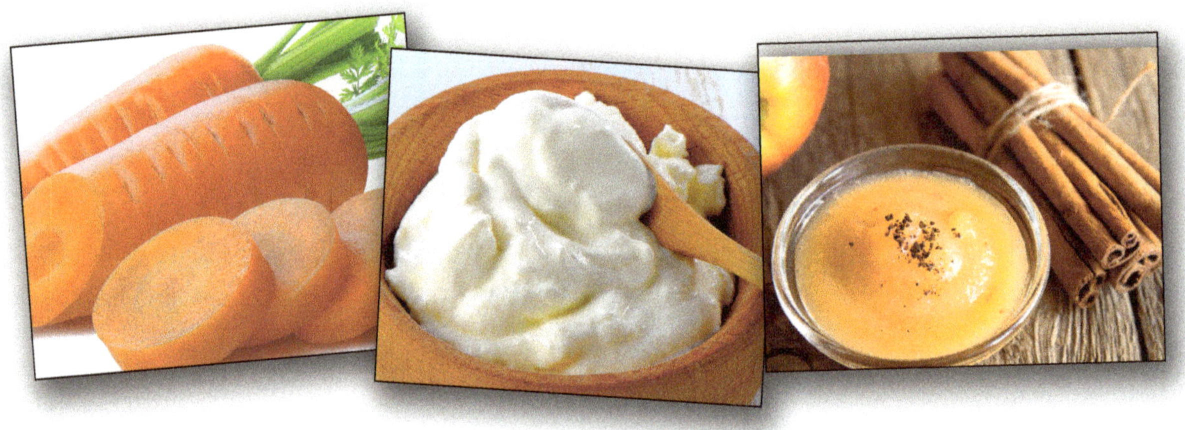

no sugar carrot cake pancakes

ingredients

½ C raisins
2 to 3 carrots
1 C plain yogurt
2 eggs (sub ½ cup puréed silken tofu)
¼ C unsweetened applesauce
1 C all-purpose flour
1½ tsp cinnamon
1 tsp baking powder
½ tsp salt
butter/olive oil/nonstick spray (for cooking)

plump+drain

Add ½ **cup of raisins** to a saucepan on your stovetop with enough water to cover about an inch above the raisins. Simmer over low heat for about 5 minutes, until the raisins have plumped and almost doubled in size. Remove from the heat and let cool. Drain the water and add the raisins to a large bowl. Let them sit and cool while you make the rest of your pancakes.

grate+mix

Have your kids grate **2 to 3 carrots** (for ½ cup grated carrot) and set to the side. Then measure and mix together **1 cup yogurt, 2 eggs**, and ¼ **cup applesauce** to the bowl with the cooled, plumped raisins. Have your kids whisk this mix vigorously until the raisins begin to fall apart. (You cannot taste the flavor or texture of the raisins. They are used to sweeten the pancakes without any processed sugars!)

combine+pour

Have your kids measure and combine the dry ingredients in a new bowl: **1 cup of flour, 1½ teaspoons of cinnamon, 1 tsp of baking powder,** and ½ **tsp of salt.** Pour the wet ingredients into the dry ingredients. Add the grated carrots to the mixture and mix with a wooden spoon only until incorporated—don't over mix!

brush+drop+flip

Heat a nonstick skillet on your stovetop over medium heat. Brush the skillet with a **touch of butter, olive oil, or nonstick spray.** Drop 1 tablespoon dollops of batter onto your preheated skillet. Cook the pancakes on the first side for about 3 to 4 minutes, until the top starts to bubble and the edges start to cook. Flip the pancakes and cook for another 3 to 4 minutes. Makes about 24 coin-sized pancakes.

FLOUR: Sift your flour before using! Sifted flour helps ensure a smooth, even texture to your baked goods.

spiced cream cheese kid-made butter

ingredients

¼ C heavy cream
pinch cinnamon
¼ C cream cheese (softened)
honey to taste

combine+shake+shake+shake!

While the pancakes are cooking, have your kids combine ¼ **cup of cream** and **a pinch of cinnamon** into a plastic container or glass jar with a tight-fitting lid and shake, shake, shake! The butter needs to be shaken for at least 5 minutes. It might seem like it will never become butter but stick with it—when you hear a "sloshing" sound (the buttermilk separating from the butter fat), you've just made butter!

drain+stir

Soften a ¼ **cup of cream cheese**. When the buttermilk and butter have separated, drain the buttermilk from the solid butter and stir the butter in with softened cream cheese and honey to taste. Top your *No Sugar Carrot Cake Pancakes* with your spiced butter and some extra honey and YUM!

Crispy Korean "Pajeon" Kid-Made Pancakes

+ Umami Sweet-Sour Soy Sauce + Iced Ginger Cinnamon Punch

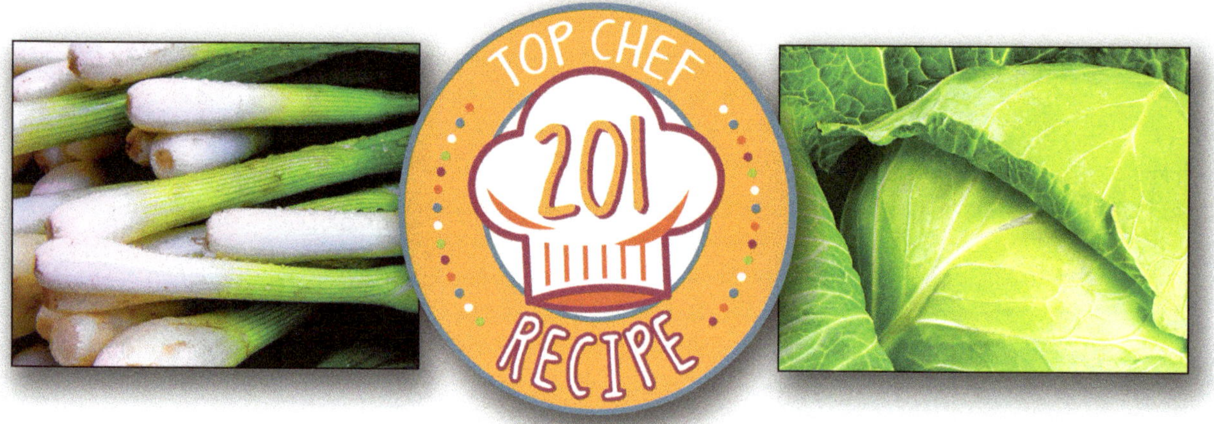

In Korean, pa means "green onion" and jeon means "fried cake." Put them together and you get a scrumptious green onion fried cake, also known as... a pancake! There are several versions of jeon in South Korea, which include kimchi, seafood, and squid! In our version, we encourage kid chefs to choose their own jeon flavorings.

add (at least !) 3 of the following ingredients to your pancakes

- 1 carrot
- 1 zucchini
- ¼ head cabbage
- 1 bell pepper
- 3 radishes
- 3 green onions
- frozen corn, peas, hashbrowns (thawed)

shred+dice+slice

Before starting, have fun choosing the ingredients you will add to your pajeon pancakes! Shred your **carrot, zucchini,** or **cabbage,** chop your **bell pepper** or **radishes** into small bits, and/or slice the **green onions**. Set to the side.

crispy korean "pajeon" kid-made pancakes

ingredients

1½ C all-purpose (sub gluten-free flour)
3 T cornstarch
½ tsp garlic powder
¾ tsp salt
1 egg
1 C ice
3 T butter or olive oil (for cooking)

measure+sift+crack+whisk

Measure and add **1½ cups of flour** to a large mixing bowl. Add **3 tablespoons of cornstarch, ½ teaspoon of garlic powder,** and **¾ teaspoon of salt.** Use a whisk to mix and sift out any lumps! Into a separate mixing bowl, crack **1 egg** and whisk it.

combine+stir+whisk

Combine **1 cup of ice** with 2 cups of water. Stir until ice melts, then measure 1½ cups of the ice-cold water and add it to the whisked egg. Whisk the ice water and egg until combined.

pour+fold

Pour the dry ingredients into the wet ingredients and fold together until all bits of flour disappear. Then add any additional ingredients you've sliced, diced, or shredded and mix gently again.

melt+fry+flip

Melt **3 tablespoons of butter or olive oil** in a large skillet over medium heat. Ladle about 2 tablespoons of batter for each pancake into your skillet. Cook for 1 minute and then flip when golden brown on one side. Cook the second side until golden brown. Continue until you've cooked all your batter, adding more butter or olive oil to the skillet between batches as needed. Serve with *Umami Sweet-Sour Dipping Sauce* and shout *Gon-Bae*, which is the Korean version of "Cheers!"

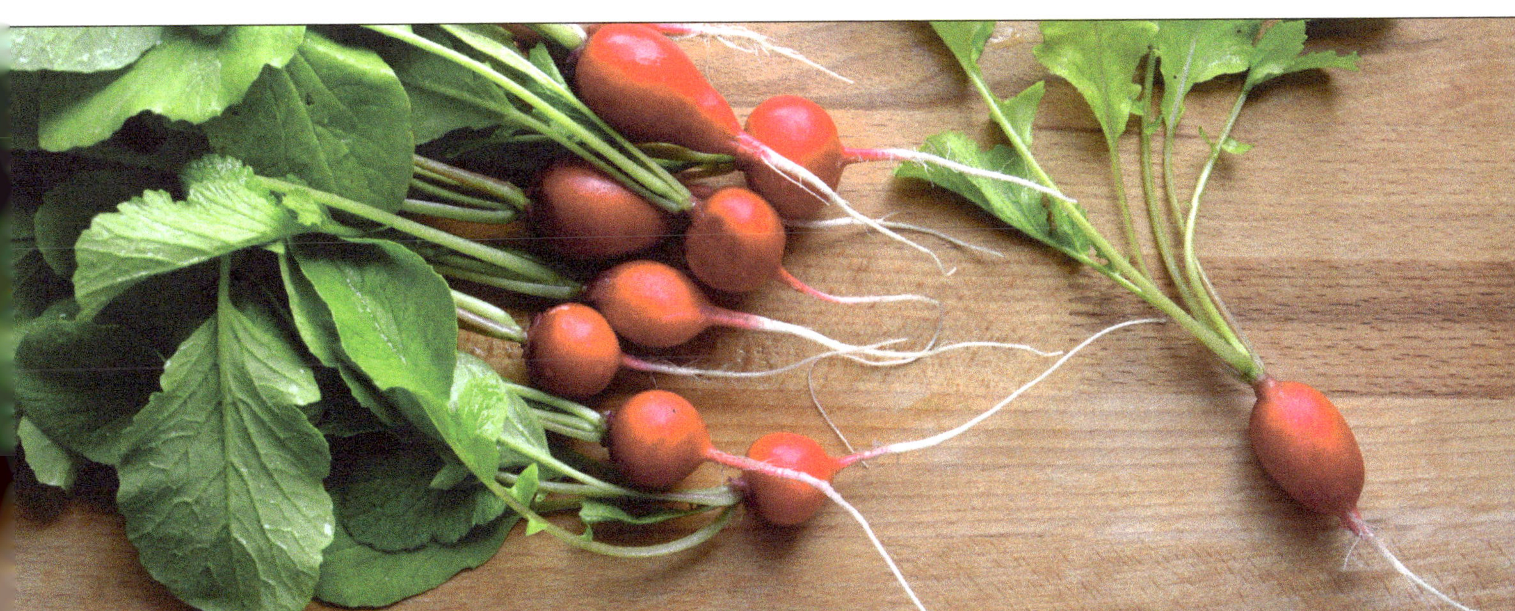

umami sweet-sour soy sauce

ingredients

1 green onion
1 garlic clove
2 T soy sauce
2 tsp white/rice wine vinegar
2 tsp toasted sesame oil
1 tsp sugar

slice+measure+whisk

Slice **1 green onion** into thin pieces and mince **1 garlic clove**. Measure and whisk together **2 tablespoons of soy sauce, 2 teaspoons of vinegar, 2 teaspoons of sesame oil, 1 teaspoon of sugar,** and **1 tablespoon water.** Stir in sliced scallions and minced garlic. Taste and adjust! Serve to dip with hot *Krispy Korean "Pajeon" Kid-Made Pancakes*!

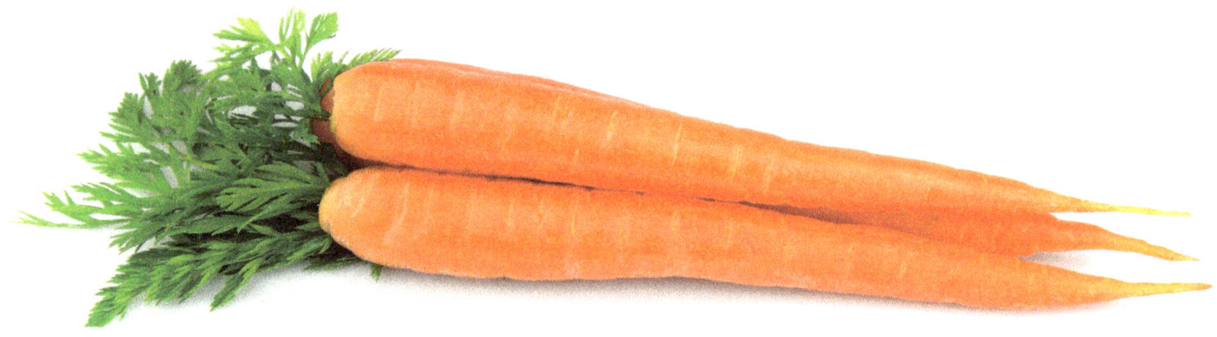

iced ginger cinnamon punch

ingredients

3 C apple juice
1-inch piece fresh ginger
1 tsp cinnamon
ice

measure+peel+slice

Measure and add **3 cups of apple juice** to a blender. Peel a **1-inch piece of ginger** using the back of a spoon. Slice ginger into thin pieces.

blend+strain+pour

Add ginger slices and **1 teaspoon of cinnamon** to the blender. Blend on high until ginger is pulverized, then strain through a sieve to catch any remaining pieces. Pour into small cups over **ice** and CHEERS!

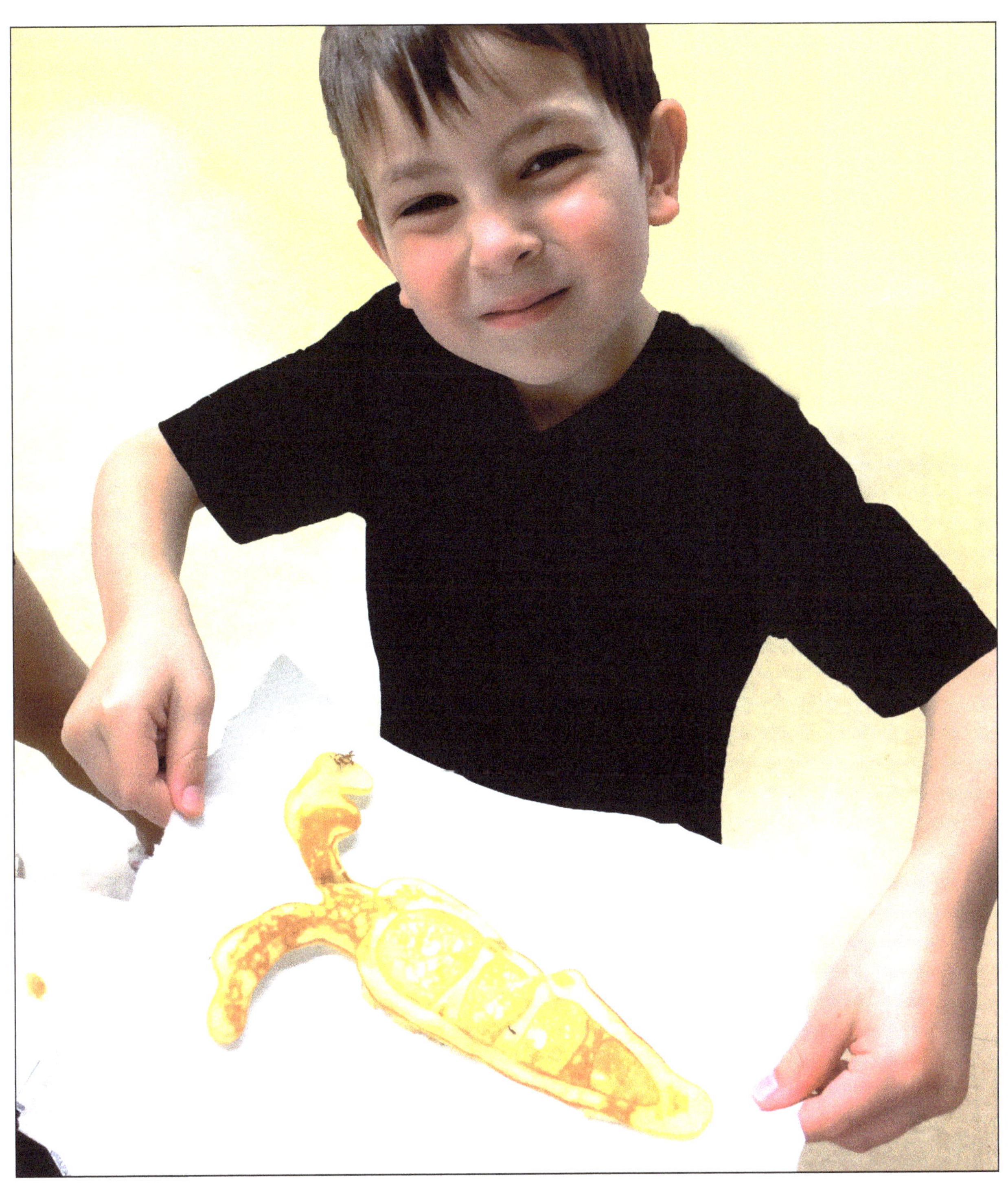

Time for a Laugh!

What did the pajeon pancake say to the other?

I'm SOY in love with you.

choose your own adventure!

UN-RECIPE!

BUTTERS + SYRUPS

butter base:

Start with **½ stick of softened butter** in a mixing bowl.
(or churn your own butter by shaking **¼ cup of heavy whipping cream** in a jar with a tight-fitting lid until you hear a sloshing sound—shake, shake, slosh!)

savory butters:

ADD SEASONING BASE!
¼ teaspoon salt + 1/8 teaspoon pepper

ADD FLAVOR!
1 teaspoon:

- dash of hot sauce
- goat cheese / cream cheese
- grated Parmesan cheese
- dill / chives / chili flakes / paprika
- mustard
- sun-dried tomatoes
- chopped olives / capers
- fresh parsley / fresh basil / chives
- lemon zest / garlic powder / onion powder

sweet butters:

SWEETNER!
1 teaspoon:

white sugar
brown sugar
agave nectar
honey
maple syrup
stevia

FLAVOR!
1 to 2 big pinches:

cinnamon
pumpkin pie spice
cocoa powder
lemon zest
sprinkles
chocolate chips
coconut flakes
dried fruits

½ teaspoon:

vanilla extract
mint extract
almond extract
apple juice
berry juice
(cooled) brewed teas

MIX IT REAL GOOD! OR WHIP IT WITH A r.

syrup base:

Start with combining **¼ cup of water** and **¼ cup of sugar** in a small saucepan.

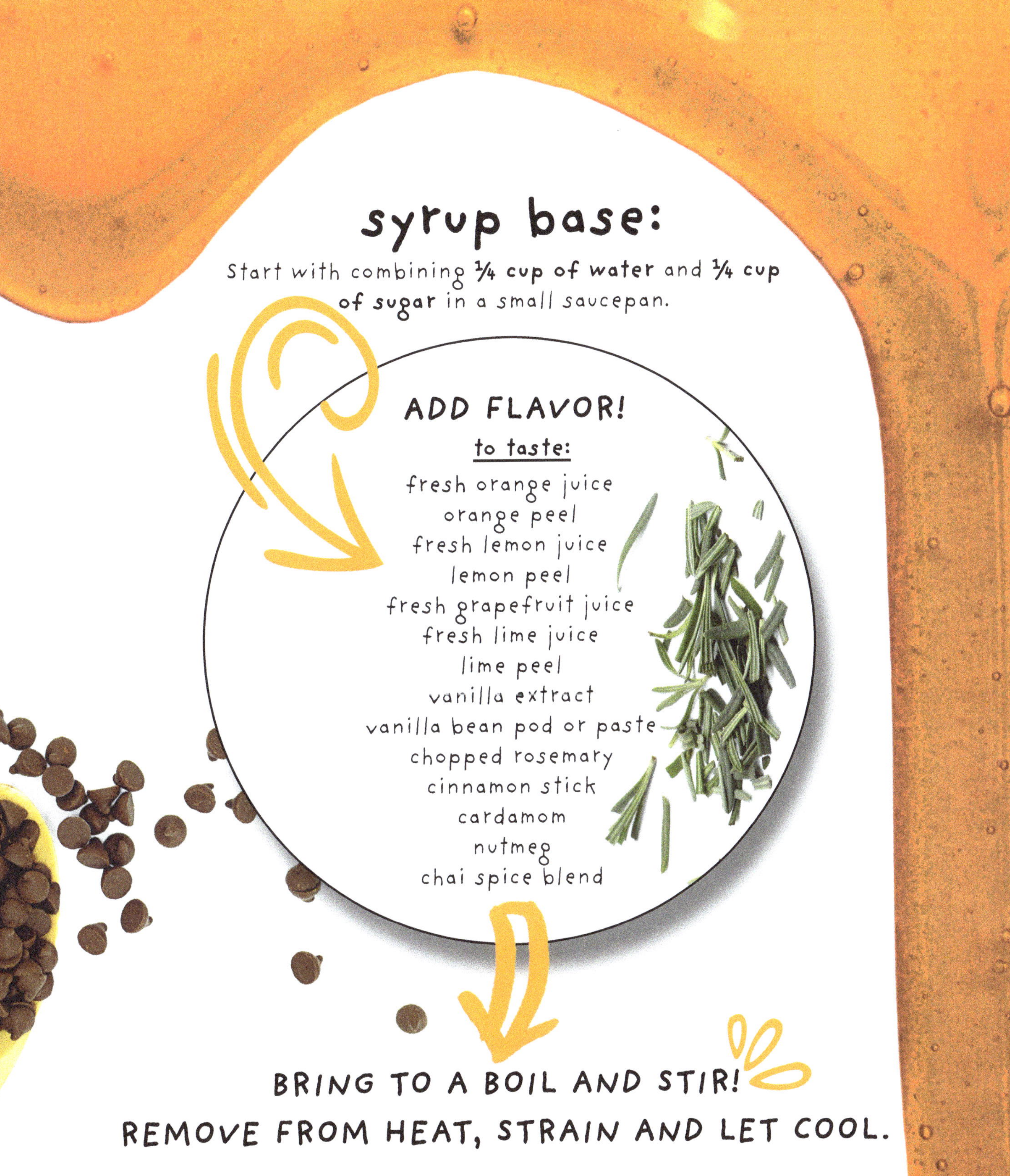

ADD FLAVOR!

to taste:

fresh orange juice
orange peel
fresh lemon juice
lemon peel
fresh grapefruit juice
fresh lime juice
lime peel
vanilla extract
vanilla bean pod or paste
chopped rosemary
cinnamon stick
cardamom
nutmeg
chai spice blend

BRING TO A BOIL AND STIR!

REMOVE FROM HEAT, STRAIN AND LET COOL.

DRIZZLE + ENJOY!

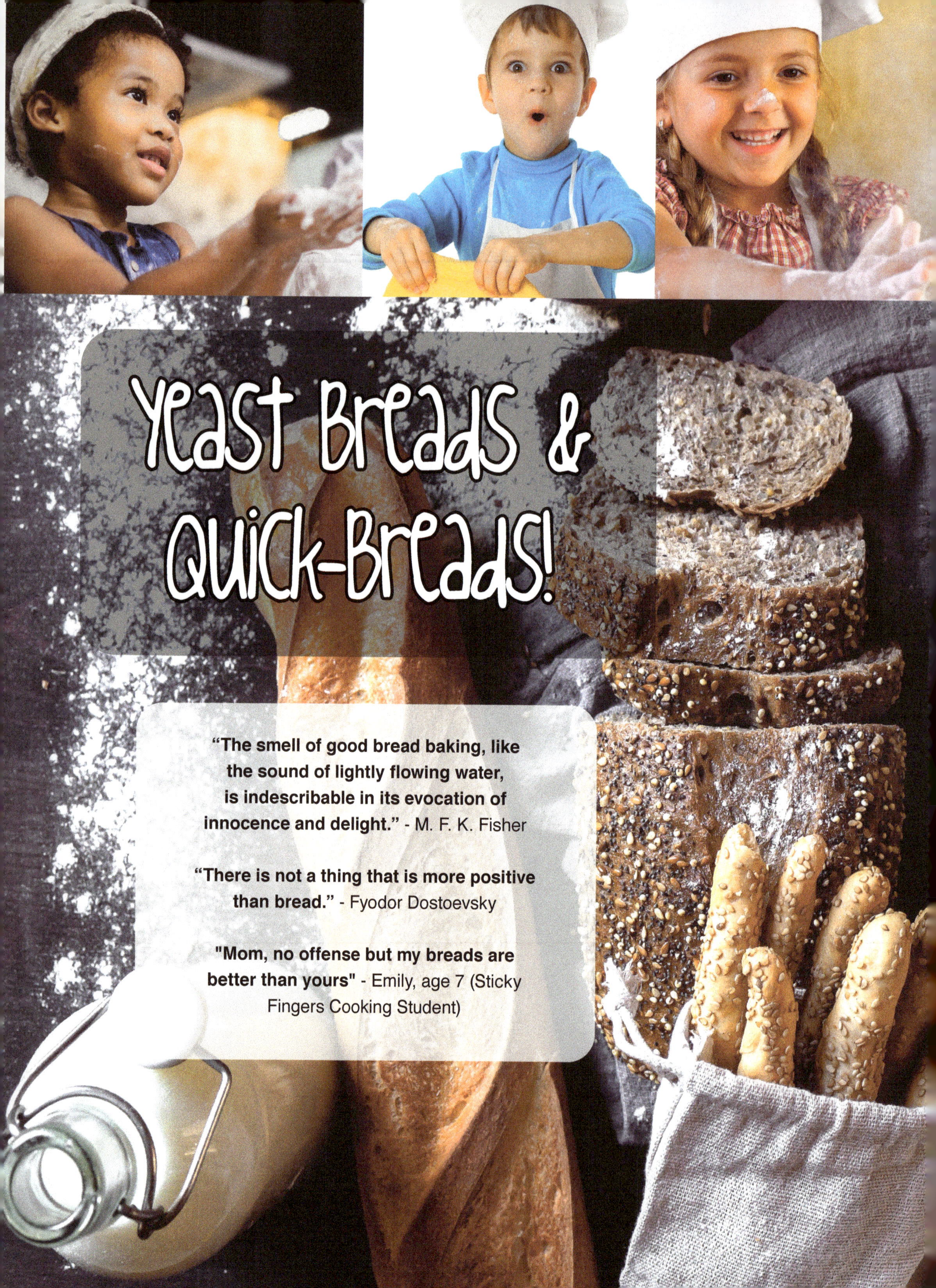

Yeast Breads & Quick-Breads!

"The smell of good bread baking, like the sound of lightly flowing water, is indescribable in its evocation of innocence and delight." - M. F. K. Fisher

"There is not a thing that is more positive than bread." - Fyodor Dostoevsky

"Mom, no offense but my breads are better than yours" - Emily, age 7 (Sticky Fingers Cooking Student)

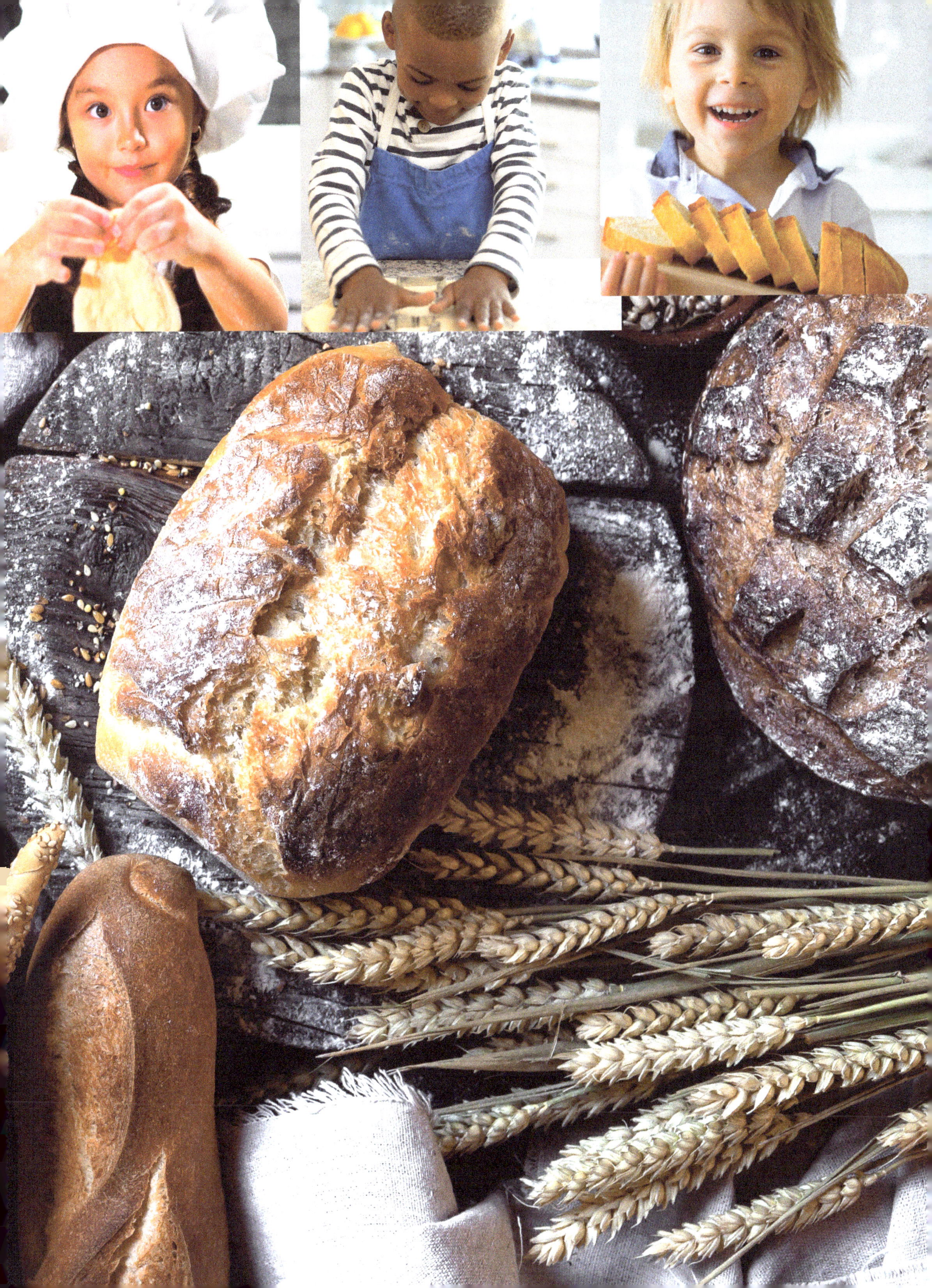

Fresh French Bread Rolls

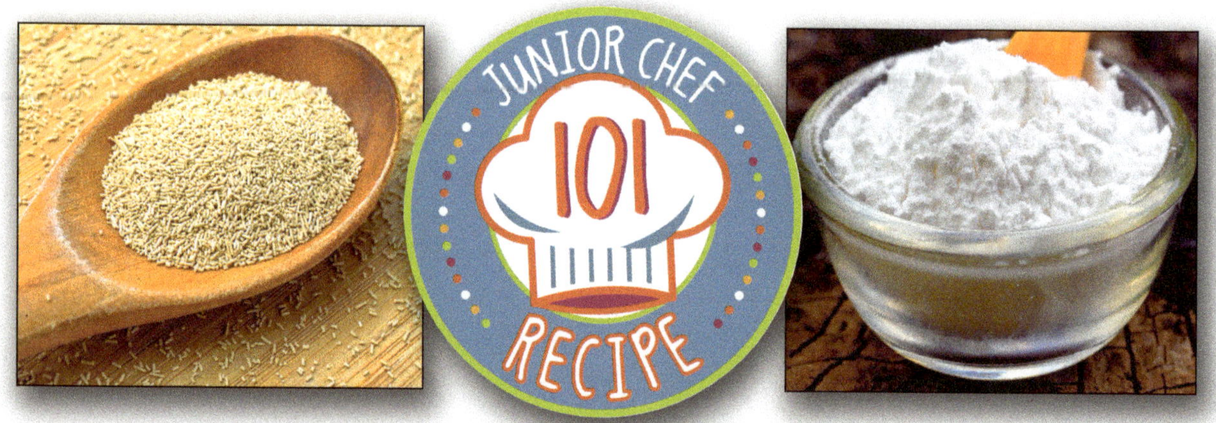

fresh french bread rolls

ingredients

1 C + 2 T warm water
⅓ C oil
2 T active dry yeast
¼ C sugar
1 egg
½ C Parmesan (or Asiago cheese)
3½ C all-purpose (or bread flour)
1 tsp salt

preheat+measure+mix+rest

Preheat oven to 400 degrees F. In a mixing bowl, measure and mix together **1 cup + 2 tablespoons of warm water, ⅓ cup of oil, 2 tablespoons of active dry yeast,** and ¼ **cup of sugar.** Allow this mixture to rest for at least 15 minutes.

crack+whisk+add

Crack **1 egg** and whisk it in a bowl. Add whisked egg to the yeast mixture. Add ½ **cup Parmesan.** Measure **3½ cups of flour** and **1 teaspoon salt** together in a separate mixing bowl. Add flour ½ cup at a time and mix well until a dough is formed.

rest+oil+bake

Let dough rest for 5 to 20 more minutes. Brush two muffin pans with oil. Then shape the dough into 24 balls and nestle one into each well of the muffin pan. Bake until bread rolls rise and are golden brown on top, about 15 to 20 minutes.

Quick Kid-made Tortillas

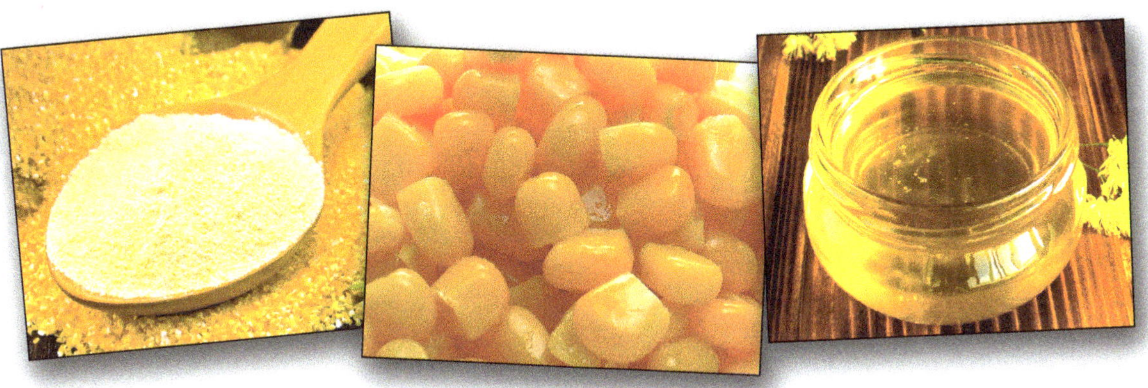

quick kid-made tortillas

ingredients

1½ C arepa flour*
¼ C frozen (thawed) corn kernels
1 tsp canola oil (+ more for cooking)
pinch salt
1½ cups warm water

**Arepa flour is a precooked corn flour and should not be confused with masa harina. Arepa flour is sold as masarepa, marina precocida, or masa al instante. It can be found in most grocery stores and Latin American groceries.*

measure+mix+cover

n a bowl, have your kids measure and mix together 1½ **cups of flour,** ¼ **cup of corn kernels, 1 teaspoon of canola oil,** and **a pinch of salt.** Pour in 1½ **cups of warm water** and mix with a spoon until the dough comes together. Cover with plastic wrap and let rest for 5 minutes.

knead+moisten

Remove the dough from the bowl and knead for about 5 minutes, having your kids moisten their clean hands and the board with sprinkles of water as they work. Kneading with additional moisture is an important step in making a tender tortilla. The dough should be smooth with no cracking around the edges, and it should be moist but not sticky.

form+cook

Have your kids form the dough into disks that are about 3 inches around and ½ inch thick. Add a few tablespoons of oil to a nonstick skillet and set stovetop to medium heat. Cook the tortillas for a few minutes on each side until a golden, crispy crust forms and the tortillas are golden brown. Remove from heat and let rest.

Scrumptiously Savory Chimichurri Monkey Bread

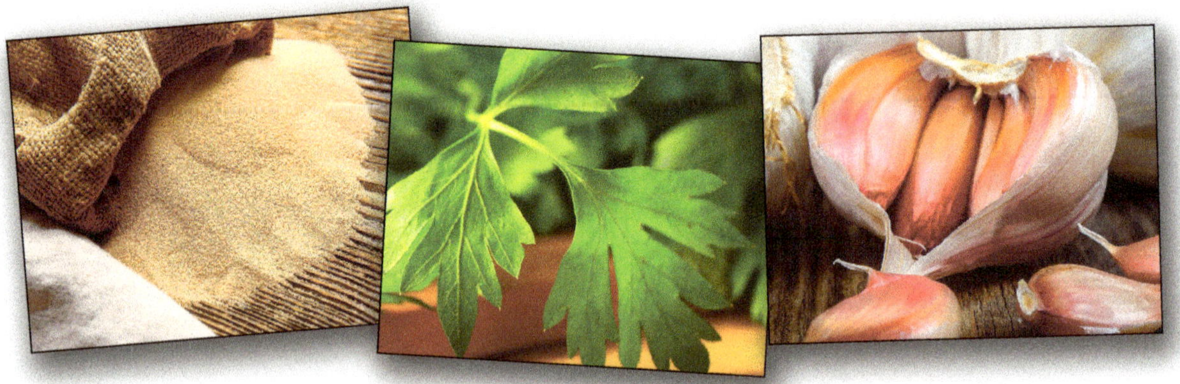

Chimichurri (CHIMmy-CHURie) is a traditional South American marinade similar to a pesto, and it's delicious as a topping on almost anything, like our monkey bread. Enjoy this bread as it is meant to be eaten… by tearing it apart with your fingers!

chimichurri sauce

ingredients

1 to 2 bunches flat-leaf parsley
1 garlic clove
2 tsp oregano
1 T red wine vinegar
1 T honey
½ tsp salt
pinch pepper
¼ C olive oil

rinse+tear+mince

First rinse **1 to 2 bunches of parsley** (you want 2 cups of packed leaves total). Save a small handful of leaves for the *Awesome Agua Fresca (recipe below!)*. Then have your kids tear the leaves from the stems and mince them to tiny pieces—the tinier the better! Add minced leaves to your blender or food processor.

crush+peel+mince

Crush **1 garlic clove** and peel it. Then mince finely and add to your blender or food processor.

measure+add

Measure **2 teaspoons of oregano, 1 tablespoon of vinegar, 1 tablespoon of honey, ½ teaspoon of salt, a pinch of pepper,** and 2 tablespoons of water and add to your blender or food processor.

pulse+stream+blend

Pulse the ingredients a few times, then stream in ¼ **cup of olive oil** while your blender or food processor purées the sauce!

scrumptiously savory monkey bread

ingredients

- 2 T warm water
- 1 tsp active dry yeast
- 2 T sugar (+ more for activating yeast)
- 2½ C all-purpose flour (+ more if needed)
- ½ tsp salt
- 1 egg
- 4 T butter
- ½ C + 2 T whole milk

preheat+measure+sprinkle+bloom

Preheat oven to 375 degrees F. Measure **2 tablespoons of warm water** with **1 teaspoon of yeast** in a small bowl and whisk. Have kids sprinkle the water and yeast with a few pinches of sugar and whisk again. Set aside to let yeast "bloom" or "wake up!"

measure+add+mix

Add **2½ cups of flour, ½ teaspoon of salt**, and **2 tablespoons of sugar** to a mixing bowl and use a whisk or a fork to mix.

crack+whisk+mix

Crack 1 egg and whisk it in a separate mixing bowl. Soften **4 tablespoons of butter**, breaking the butter up into individual tablespoons to make it easier to mix. Then add ½ **cup + 2 tablespoons of milk** to the egg and butter and mix well. Then, add yeast/water mixture and mix again.

mix+knead+add

Mix dry ingredients into wet ingredients with a wooden spoon. Using clean hands, knead the dough in the bowl, adding more flour by the tablespoon if dough is too sticky (dough should be somewhat sticky, but not so much that it completely sticks to your hands).

tear+roll+add+bake

Tear off small chunks of dough and roll them into golf ball-sized chunks, adding sprinkles of flour if dough is still too sticky. Add dough balls to a big mixing bowl with ½ cup of *Chimichurri Sauce* and toss with hands until balls are evenly coated (save the rest for dipping!) Place 2 to 3 dough balls into each well of a muffin pan and bake for 25 to 35 minutes, or until bread is golden brown on the surface and dough is cooked through. Serve with extra *Chimichurri Sauce* for extra YUM!

Easy Irish Soda Bread Biscuits

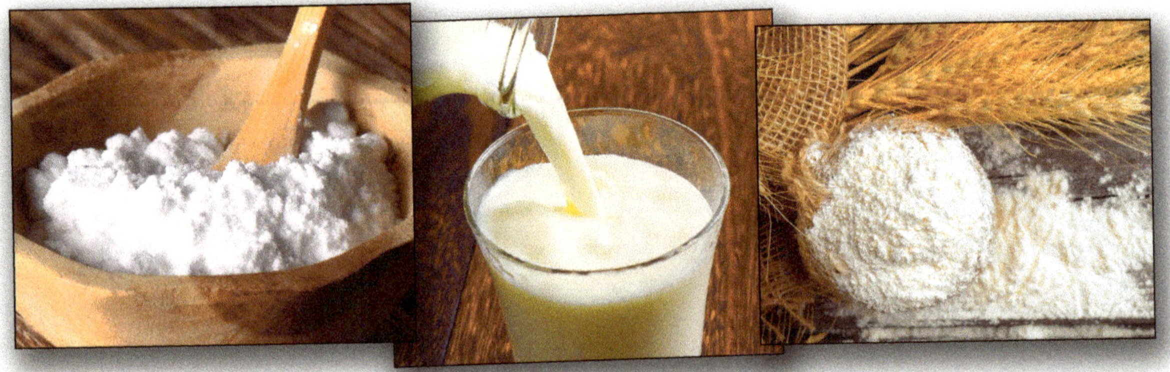

The four key components of any Irish soda bread are flour, salt, buttermilk, and... baking soda, of course! Since the bread contains no yeast, it instead relies on gas bubbles produced from the baking soda reacting with our quick, homemade buttermilk (yes, you can make your own buttermilk!). Our bread is an easy and tasty demonstration of why baking is a science!

easy irish soda bread biscuits

ingredients

- 2¼ C all-purpose flour
- ⅓ C sugar
- ¼ tsp baking soda
- 2 tsp baking powder
- 1 tsp caraway seeds
- ½ tsp salt
- 1 C milk
- 1 T lemon juice
- ¼ C butter
- 1 egg
- ¼ C olive oil
- ½ C raisins

combine+rest+whisk

In a large bowl, measure and combine 2¼ **cups of flour, ⅓ cup of sugar, ¼ teaspoon of baking soda, 2 teaspoons of baking powder, 1 teaspoon of caraway seeds, and ½ teaspoon of salt.** In a separate bowl, combine **1 cup of milk with 1 tablespoon of lemon juice.** Let milk and lemon juice sit for 5 minutes to curdle. Then melt and add ¼ **cup of butter** and add **1 egg** and whisk again. Add ¼ **cup of olive oil** and ½ **cup of raisins** and whisk once more. Make sure you wash your hands after cracking the egg!

EGGS: Crack your eggs into a separate bowl first! That way you can scoop out any eggshells that might have fallen in before adding your eggs into your baking mixture.

preheat+mix+bake

Preheat your oven to 400 degrees F. Grease a muffin pan. Add the dry ingredients ½ cup at a time to the wet ingredients and mix well until a thick batter is formed. Divide the batter between the muffin wells, filling them ½ full. Bake until biscuits are cooked through, about 15 to 20 minutes. Spread with butter and ENJOY!

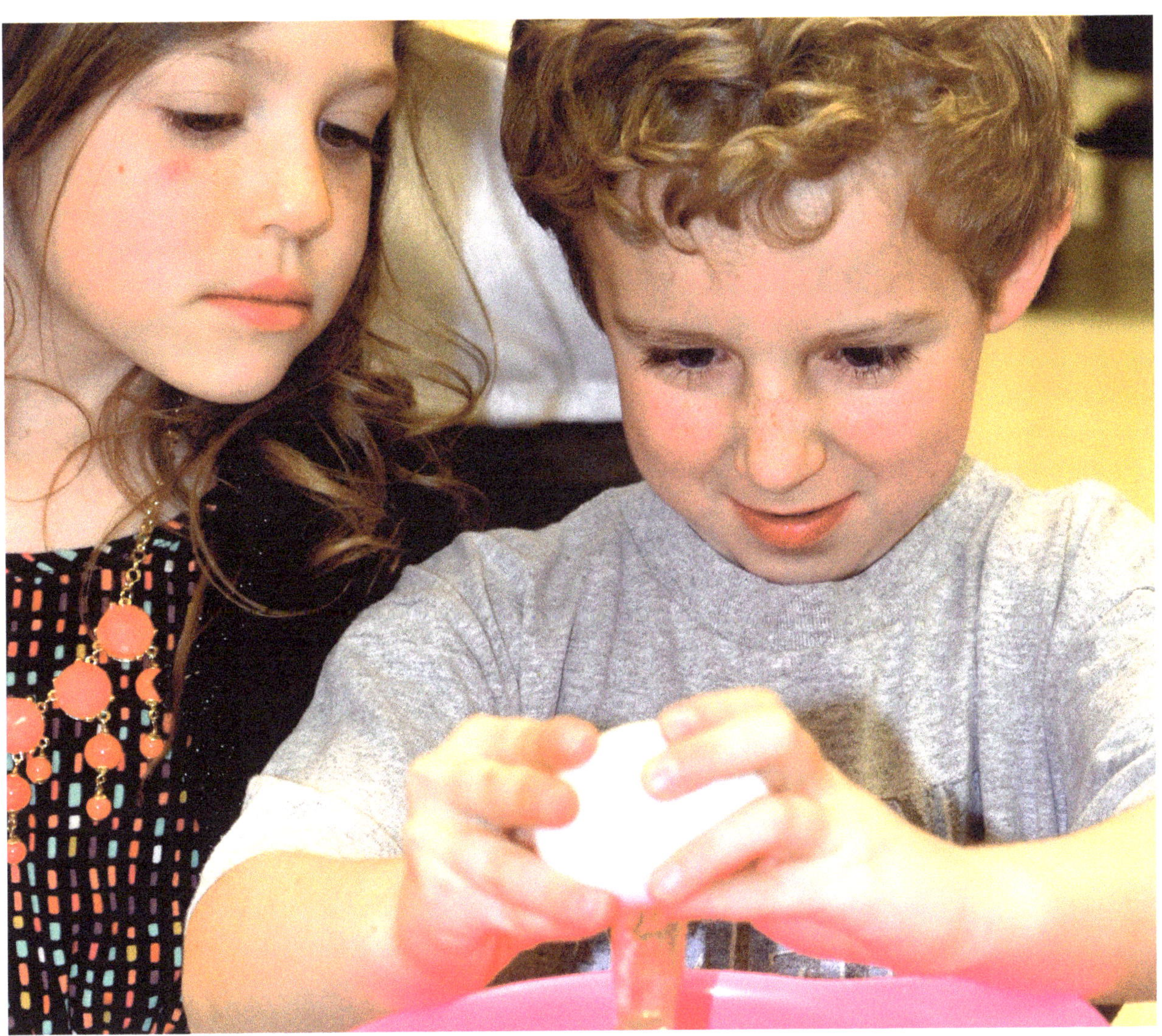

Time for a Laugh!

What did the baking soda say when the buttermilk was trying to make it angry?

You're just trying to get a rise out of me!

Apple Carrot Raisin Challah Knots
+ Pomegranate Juice Icing

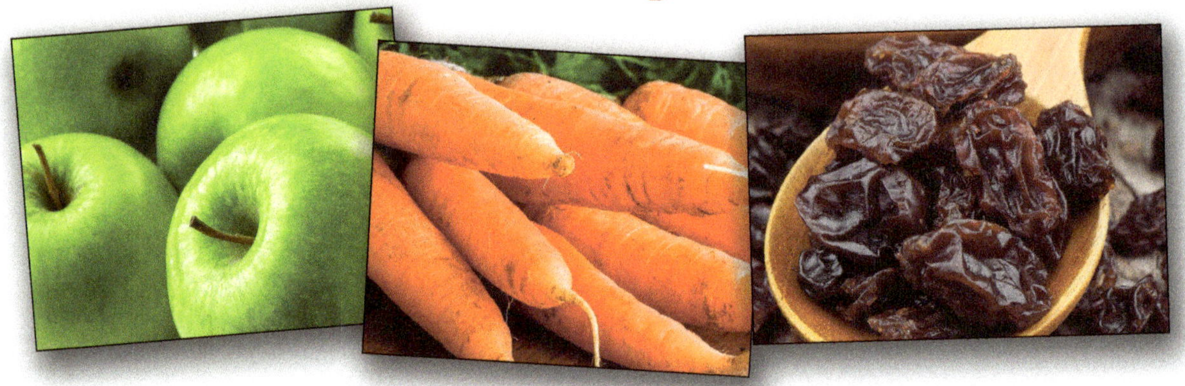

Challah (HALL-uh) is a Jewish bread that is traditionally braided or twisted, glazed with an egg wash, and sprinkled with sesame or poppy seeds. We are kicking it up a notch by adding an oh-so-good pomegranate icing to achieve that same shine and complement the addition of apples and carrot.

apple carrot raisin challah knots

ingredients

2 eggs
2 Granny Smith apples
1 large carrot
2 T unsalted butter
⅛ tsp cinnamon
⅛ tsp cardamom
¼ C raisins
2 C all-purpose flour
2 tsp baking powder
1 tsp sea salt
½ tsp baking soda
1 T sugar
2 C buttermilk
cooking spray, butter, or oil (for greasing pan)
sesame or poppy seeds (optional)

crack+beat

Start with **2 eggs**. Crack and separate the egg whites from the egg yolks, reserving the yolks. In a clean bowl, beat the egg whites with your electric mixer until they can hold a stiff peak. Set aside.

slice+grate

Have kids peel the skin off **2 apples** then chop them into small bits. Grate **1 carrot** then add apples, carrots, and **2 tablespoons of butter** to a skillet and sauté over medium heat. Add ⅛ **teaspoon of cinnamon** and ⅛ **teaspoon of cardamom** to the skillet. Sauté until the apples and carrots are soft and the spices are fragrant (about 3 to 5 minutes). Now, stir in ¼ **cup of raisins** and let cool off to the side.

mix+fold+bake

Preheat your oven to 350 degrees F. This is a good time to spray the muffin pan with cooking spray or rub it down with butter or oil. Have kids measure and mix **2 cups of flour, 2 teaspoons of baking powder, 1 teaspoon of salt, ½ teaspoon of baking soda, 1 tablespoon of sugar,** and **2 cups of buttermilk**. Add the reserved egg yolks one at a time into the buttermilk and flour mixture and beat with a whisk until smooth. Add the sautéed carrots and apples. Have kids gently fold in the egg whites into the batter. We like to let the batter sit for a few minutes at this point. Spoon the batter into the greased muffin pan wells, about 2 heaping spoonfuls each. Bake for about 10 to 15 minutes or until cooked through.

pomegranate juice icing

ingredients

1¼ C powdered sugar

2 to 3 T fresh pomegranate juice

whisk+eat

As the Challah bakes and cools, it is time to make the Pomegranate Juice Icing! Have kids measure and mix **1¼ cup of powdered suga**r and **2 to 3 tablespoons of pomegranate juice** into a medium sized bowl. Whisk and set aside. After the *Apple Carrot Raisin Challah Knots* cool for a bit pluck them out of the muffin pan, drizzle them with pomegranate juice icing, and top them with **sesame or poppy seeds**, if you like!

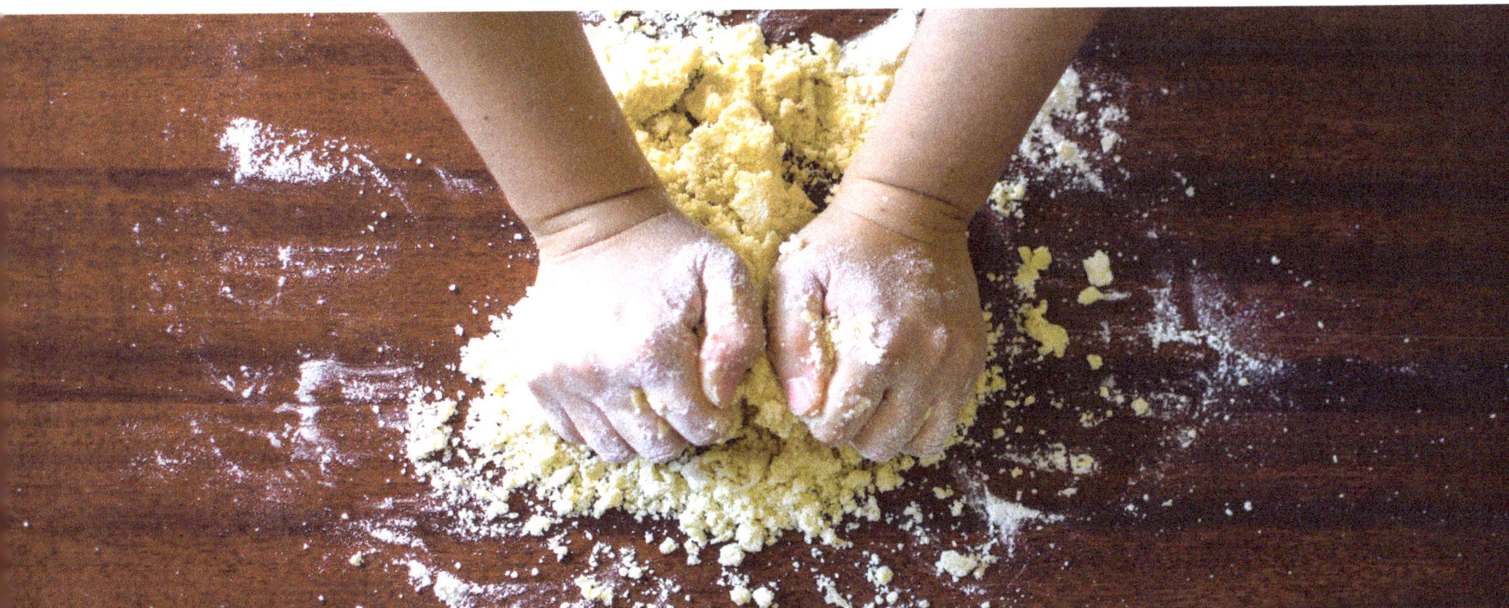

Fabulous Fast-Fresh Garlic Knots

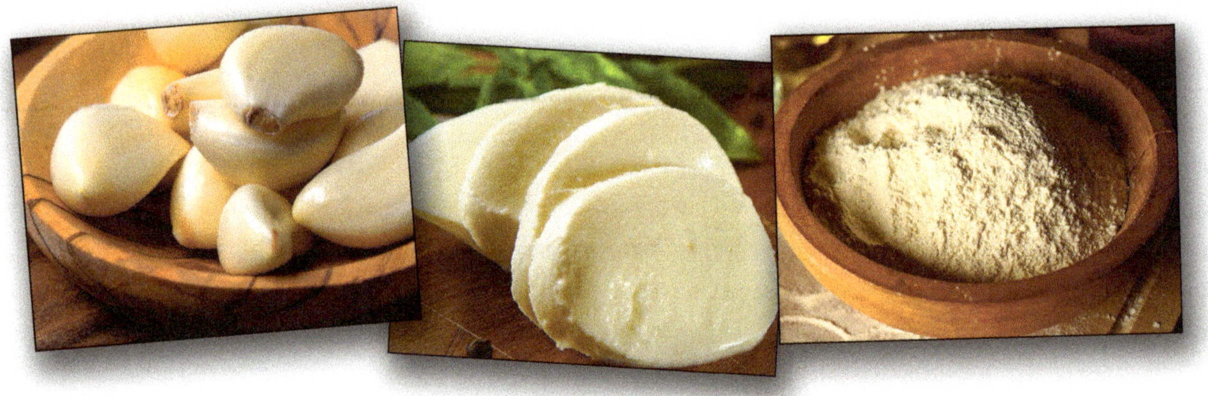

fabulous fast-fresh garlic knots

ingredients

butter or oil (for greasing pan)
1 C + 2 T warm water
1/3 C oil
2 T active dry yeast
¼ C sugar
1 egg
½ to ¾ Parmesan or mozzarella cheese
1 garlic clove
3½ all-purpose flour
1 tsp salt

preheat

Preheat your oven to 375 degrees F and grease your muffin pan with **butter or oil**.

pour+rest

In a bowl, have kids pour **1 cup + 2 tablespoons of warm water, 1/3 cup of oil, 2 tablespoons of yeast**, and **¼ cup of sugar.**

crack+whip+dice

Then, crack **1 egg** and whip the egg with the yeast mixture. Add **½ to ¾ cup Parmesan or mozzarella cheese** and have kids mince **1 garlic clove** and it to the yeast mixture and stir well.

mix+measure

In a separate small bowl, have kids mix and measure **3½ cups of flour** and **1 teaspoon of salt.** Add flour, ½ a cup at a time to the yeast mixture and mix well until a dough forms.

shape+bake

Have kids shape the dough into about 24 balls and let the dough rest for at least 20, up to 60 minutes. The more time the dough has to rise, the better! Place the dough into your greased muffin pan and bake for 15 to 20 minutes or until tops are just golden brown.

BREADS: Double check your yeast beforehand! Some yeasts are "fast-acting" or "instant" and will rise quickly while others might take much longer.

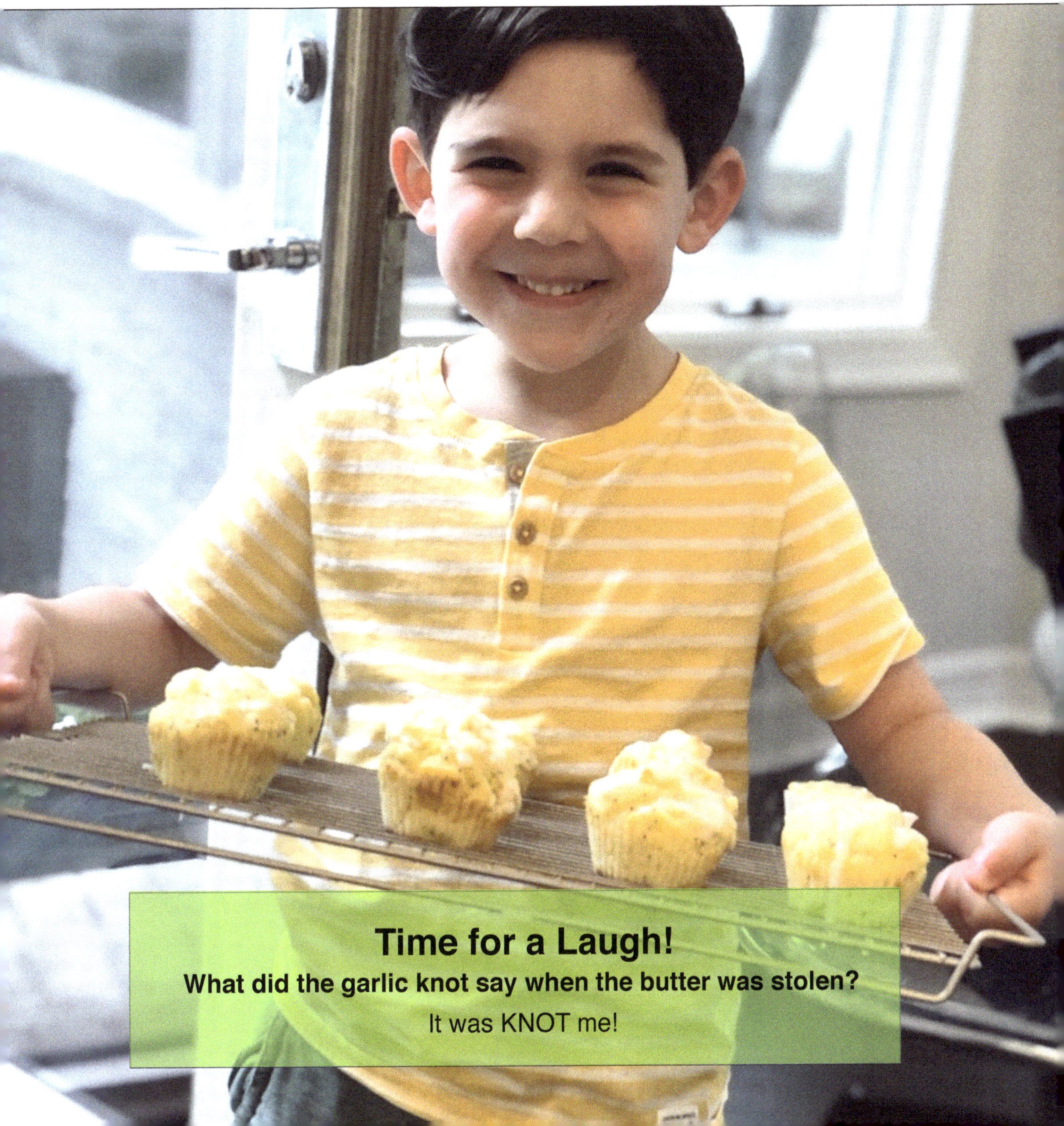

Time for a Laugh!

What did the garlic knot say when the butter was stolen?

It was KNOT me!

Ethiopian Injera Bread + Spiced Cauliflower Dip + Sparking Honey Water

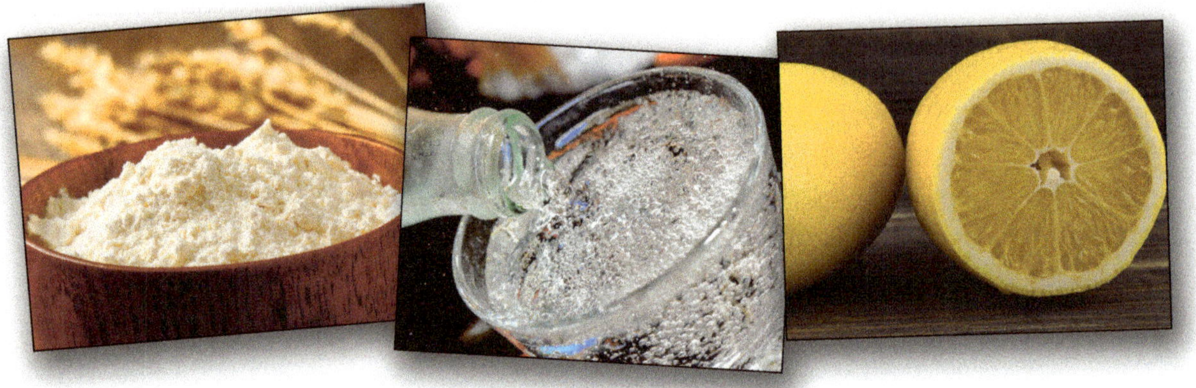

Injera (in-GEER-ra) bread is traditionally made with fermented teff, a very nutritious Ethiopian grain. To eat this crepe-like flatbread, tear a piece off with your hands and scoop up your favorite dip or roll your food inside the bread—no utensils needed!

ethiopian injera bread

ingredients

1½ C all-purpose flour
1½ T baking powder
1 tsp salt
2 to 2½ c club soda
1 T white wine vinegar
some oil (for cooking)
2 fresh lemons

measure+mix

Have kids measure and mix **1½ cups of flour, ½ tablespoons of baking powder,** and **1 teaspoon of salt** in a large bowl.

pour+stir+whisk+preheat

In the same bowl whisk **2 to 2½ cups of club soda** and **1 tablespoon of vinegar** until smooth. The consistency should be thin and pourable, like pancake batter. Set the batter aside for 10 minutes to rest. Dab a paper towel with **some oil** and rub on a nonstick skillet, then set the skillet on the stove over medium heat to preheat.

flip+cook

Ladle about ½ a cup of the batter into the skillet and spread it out with a spatula to make a large, thin crepe. Let the crepe bake in the skillet until the bubbles on the top burst and begin to dry out, about 2 to 3 minutes. Make sure to flip and cook evenly on both sides, making sure not to brown the injera too much. Continue cooking the injera until the batter runs out, wiping the skillet clean with a paper towel with each new crepe.

squeeze+brush

While you are cooking the injera, have your kids squeeze the juice from 2 lemons into a small bowl. Using a basting brush, lightly cover each injera bread with lemon juice for extra ZING! Serve immediately while it's still warm, with the Ethiopian Lemon Cauliflower Bean Dip – hands only, no silverware!

spiced califlower dip

ingredients

1 C cauliflower
1 C canned garbanzo or cannellini beans (rinsed and drained)
1 to 2 garlic cloves
2 T extra virgin olive oil
pinches of Mitmita spice blend

chop+juice

Have kids measure chop up 1 cup of cauliflower into small bits. Peel and chop 1 garlic clove and 2 tablespoons of lemon juice. Add the chopped cauliflower and the lemon juice to your blender.

throw+blend

Into the blender add 1 cup of garbanzo bans or cannellini beans, 2 tablespoons of olive oil, ½ teaspoon of salt, ½ teaspoon of pepper, and a few pinches of Mitmita spice blend. Process the dip in your blender with the lid on until smooth. Scrape down the sides as needed..

taste+serve

Taste the dip and add more salt, pepper, and/or lemon, if needed. Keep in mind that flavors of the dip will continue to intensify as it sits. Pour the dip into a serving bowl with a big drizzle of olive oil, more of the Mitmita spice blend, and a little more salt and/or pepper. If needed, adjust the seasonings again before serving with the yummy Injera Bread!

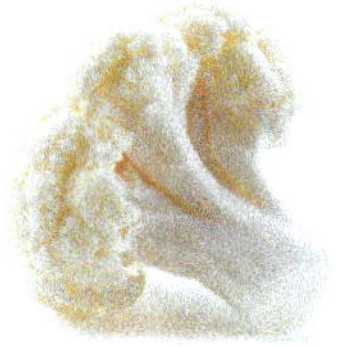
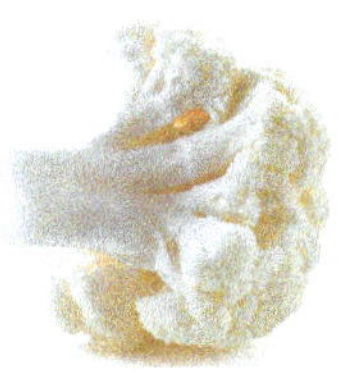
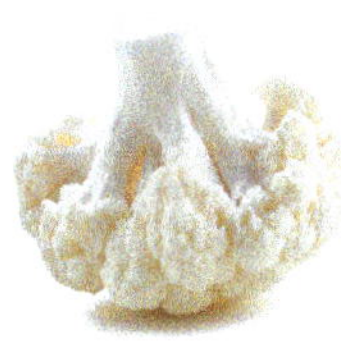
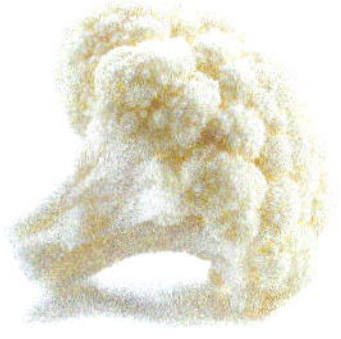
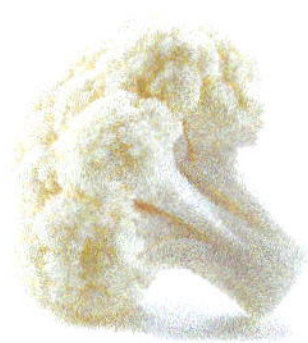
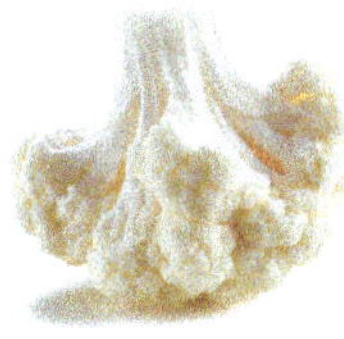

sparkling honey water

ingredients

8 T honey
2 C hot water
2 C club soda
4 T fresh lemon juice
small pinch Mitmita spice blend
ice

squeeze+stir+serve

In a pitcher, carefully stir in **8 tablespoons of honey** into **2 cups of hot water** to melt the honey and stir well. Add **2 cups of club soda, 4 tablespoons of fresh lemon juice** and a **tiny pinch of Mitmita**. Stir the ingredients together and serve in tall glasses over ice.

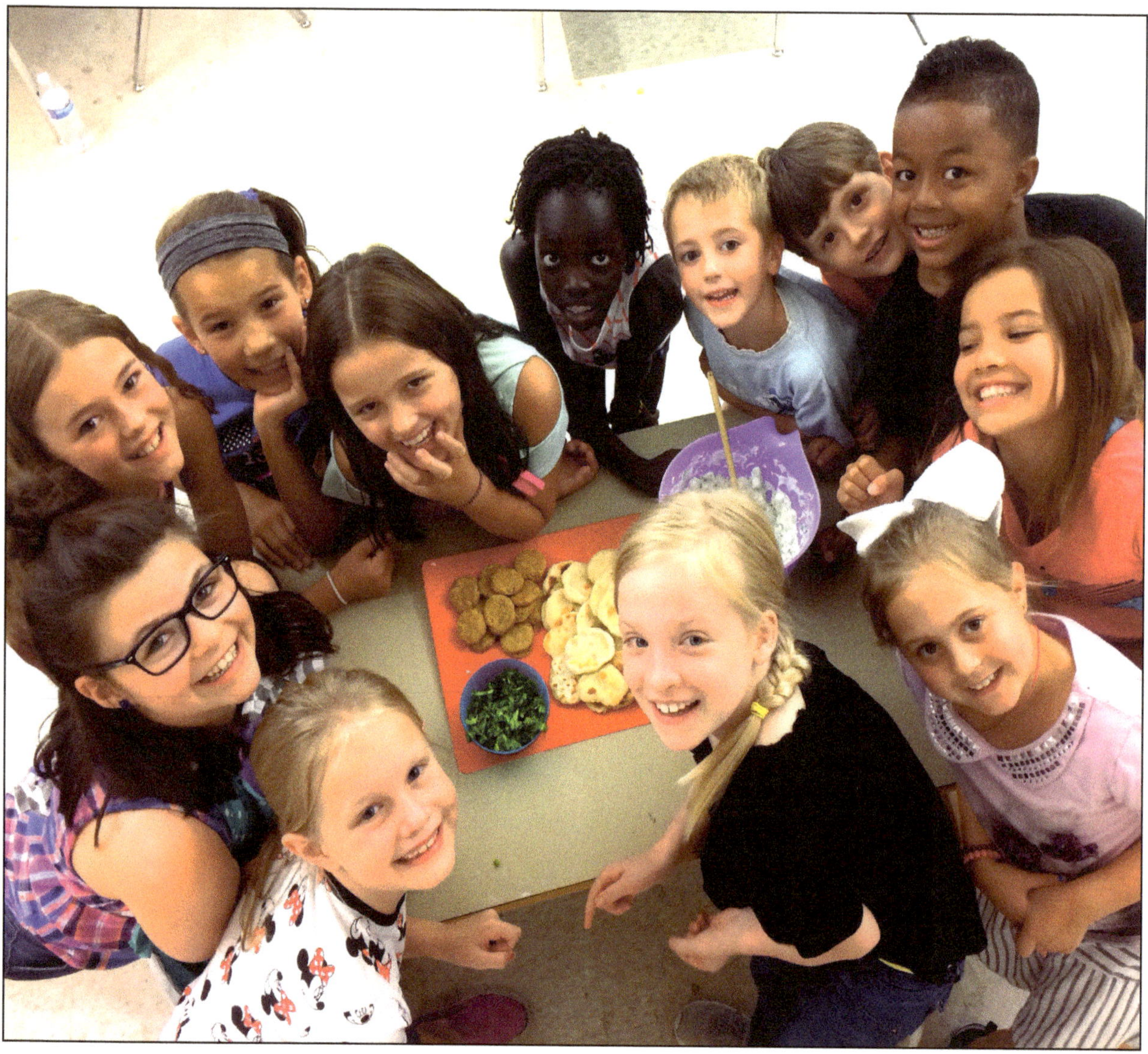

Ukranian Molasses Quick Bread

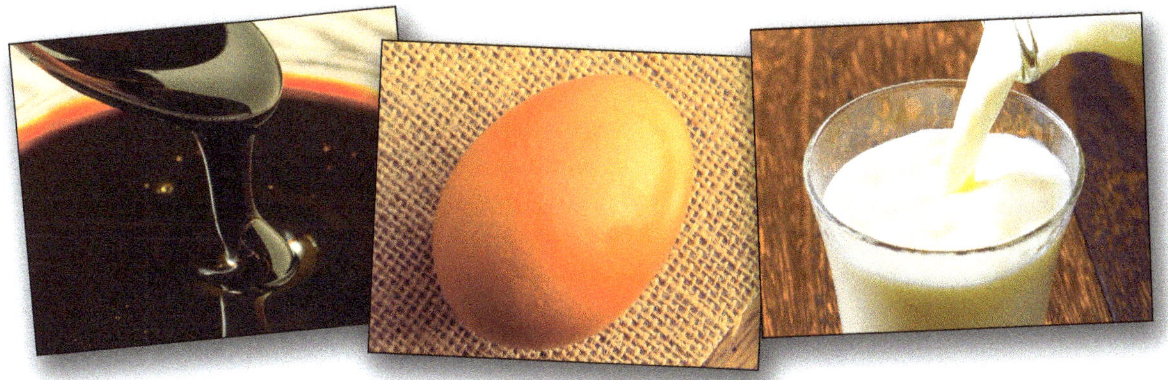

ukranian molasses quick bread

ingredients

2 C whole wheat flour
1 tsp baking powder
1 tsp baking soda
1 tsp salt
1 large egg
2 C buttermilk
3 T molasses
1½ T oil

preheat+mix+measure

Preheat oven to 350 degrees F. In a mixing bowl, have your kids mix **2 cups of whole wheat flour, 1 teaspoon of baking powder, 1 teaspoon of baking soda,** and **1 teaspoon of salt** in a medium bowl for your dry ingredients.

crack+stir

In a separate mixing bowl for your dry ingredients, crack and beat **1 egg**. Then stir in **2 cups of buttermilk, 3 tablespoons of molasses,** and **1½ tablespoons of oil** with the egg. Then stir dry mix into the wet mix.

mix+bake

Mix the dough until it just comes together. Scrape batter into a lined or greased muffin pan and bake for 10 to 15 minutes, or until the bread looks browned and a tester toothpick comes out clean. Remove the bread from the oven and set aside to cool.

Brazilian Pão de Queijo Puffs

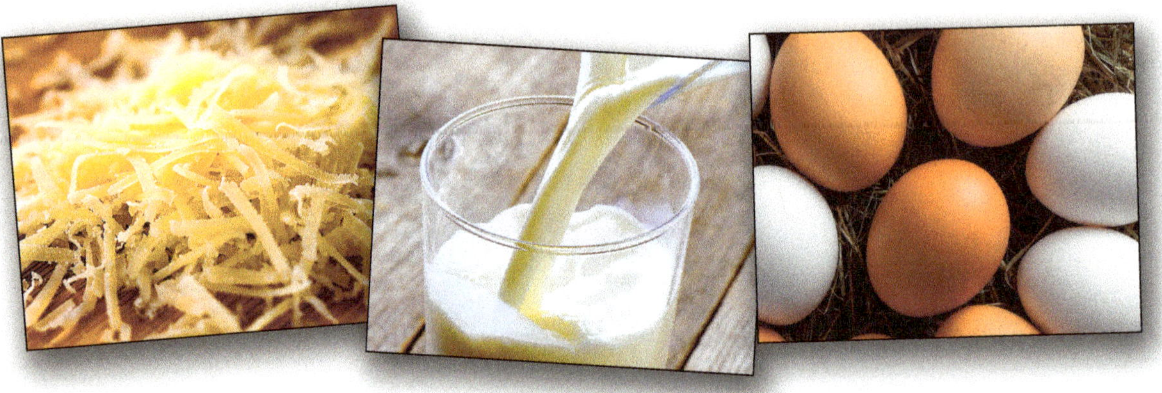

Pão de Queijo (POW de Kay-jew) translates to "bread of cheese" in Portuguese and is a popular snack or breakfast in Brazil. The dish was originally made with cassava root and then cheese was added later on. These cheesy, chewy puffs are insanely delicious and easy to make!

brazilian pão de queijo puffs

ingredients

olive oil (for greasing)
1 C whole milk
½ C vegetable oil
½ tsp salt
2 C tapioca flour
2 eggs
½ to 1 C Parmesan cheese

egg-free Brazilian pão de queijo puffs:
olive oil (for greasing)
¾ C whole milk
8 T butter
½ tsp salt
2 C tapioca flour
1 T baking powder
½ to 1 C Parmesan cheese

oil+preheat

Preheat oven to 425 degrees F. Spread a drizzle of **olive oil** inside each well of your muffin sheet.

measure+mix

In a large bowl measure and mix together **1 cup of milk, ½ cup of vegetable oil, ½ teaspoon of salt, 2 cups of flour,** and **2 eggs.** Have kids grate **½ to 1 cup of Parmesan cheese** and add to the bowl. Using a hand mixer or immersion blender, blend until smooth. Stop occasionally to scrape down the sides of the bowl with a spatula so that everything gets blended well. (At this point, you can store the batter in your fridge for up to a week!).

fill+bake

Fill your prepared muffin wells with about 2 tablespoons of batter for each bread bite. Bake in preheated oven for about 20 minutes, until puffs get puffy and lightly brown. Remove from the oven and let cool for a few minutes. Eat while warm! Note: *Pão de Queijo* is very chewy, much like Japanese mochi.

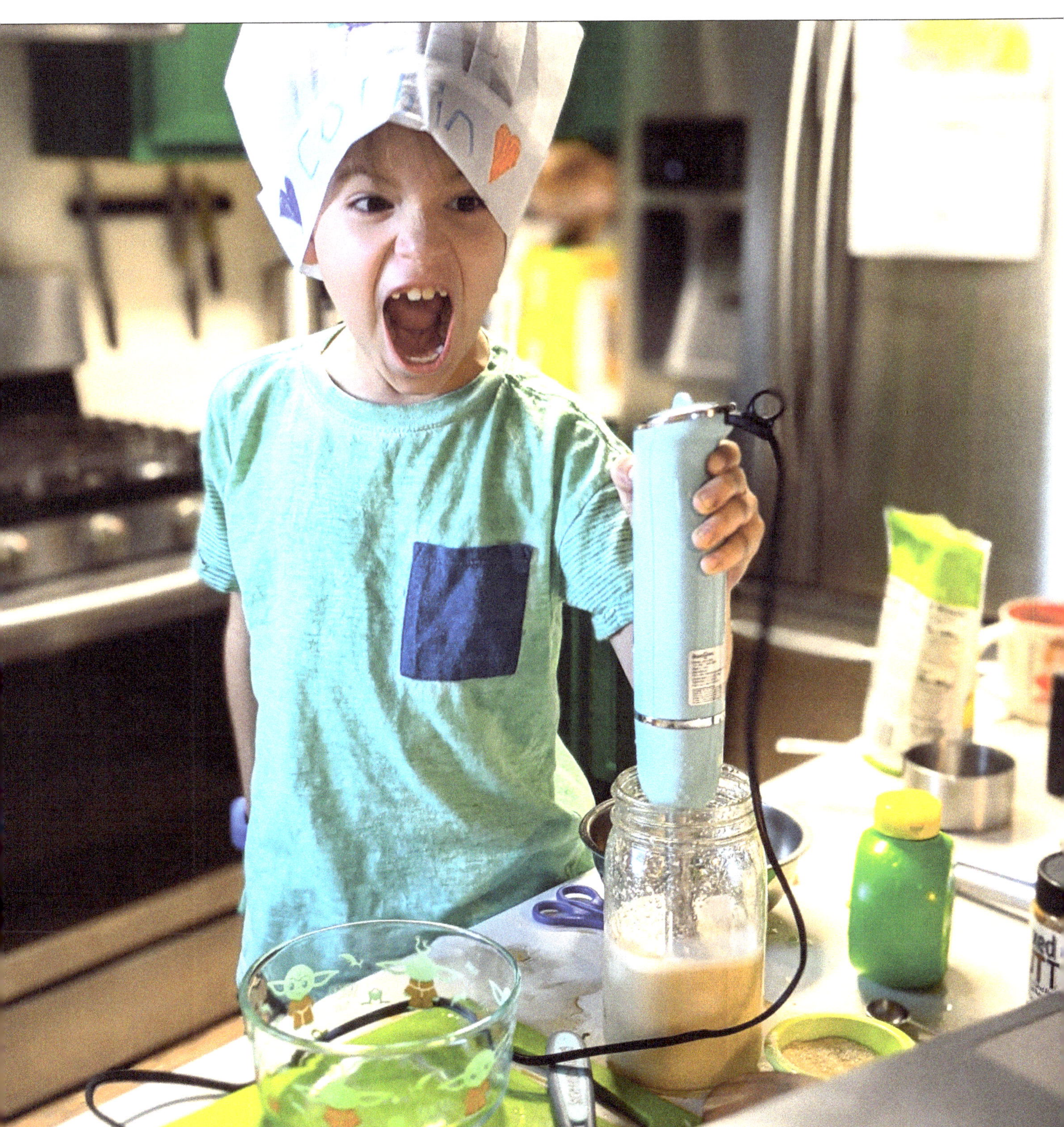

Great Grecian Personal Pan Pizzas

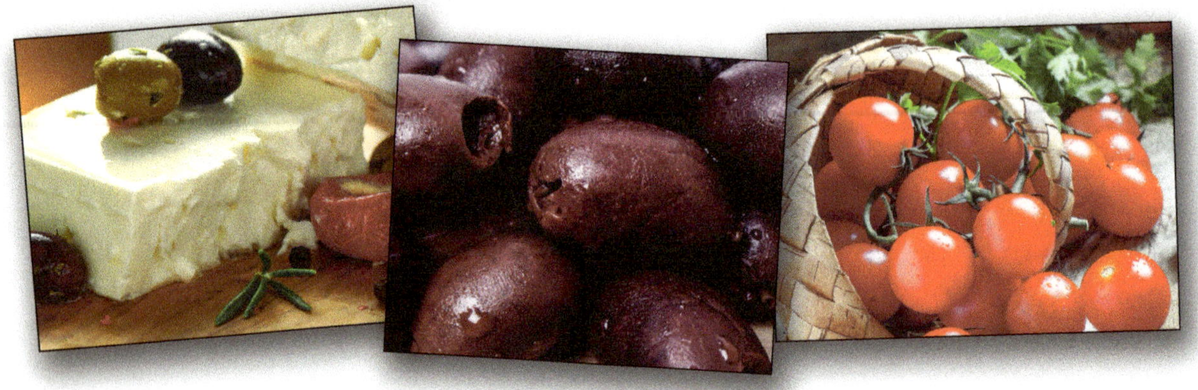

let's make pizza dough!

ingredients

2 C all-purpose flour
1 T baking powder
½ tsp salt
2 C full-fat Greek yogurt

preheat+measure+combine+whisk

Preheat oven to 400 degrees F. Measure **2 cups of flour, 1 tablespoon of baking powder,** and ½ **teaspoon of salt** in a large mixing bowl. Whisk to combine!

measure+add+stir+knead

Add **2 cups of yogurt** to the flour and use a spatula to stir. Using clean hands, kids can mix and knead the dough, incorporating the yogurt and flour together. Hands are the best way! The dough will come together quickly and easily in the mixing bowl. The dough should be soft, supple, and pliable but not sticky. Your dough should feel like soft play—dough! In really humid climates more flour may be needed. If the dough is still sticky, add more flour by the tablespoon while kneading until the texture is just right. Form dough into one big ball, cover with a damp towel, and set aside.

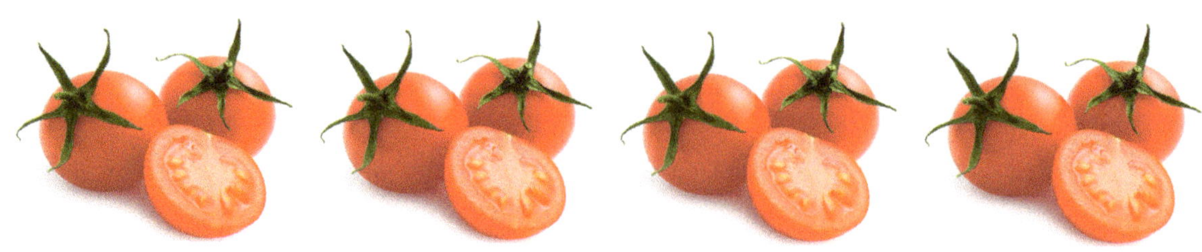

pizza sauce time!

ingredients

8 oz canned tomato sauce
2 tsp garlic powder
1 T olive oil (+ more for greasing pan)
½ tsp oregano (optional)

pour+measure+mix

Pour **8 ounces of tomato sauce** into a clean mixing bowl and add **2 teaspoons of garlic powder, 1 tablespoon of olive oil,** and **an optional ½ teaspoon of oregano** and mix! Set sauce aside.

chop the toppings!

ingredients

canned artichoke hearts (drained)
3 green onions
1 C cherry tomatoes
handful kalamata olives (pitted)
frozen (thawed) spinach
1 tsp oregano
mozzarella cheese
feta cheese

pour+measure+mix

Slice, drain and chop the **artichoke hearts** and **3 green onions** into bite-sized pieces. Chop **a handful of olives** into tiny pieces and slice **1 cup of tomatoes** into halves. Put sliced and chopped veggies into separate bowls.

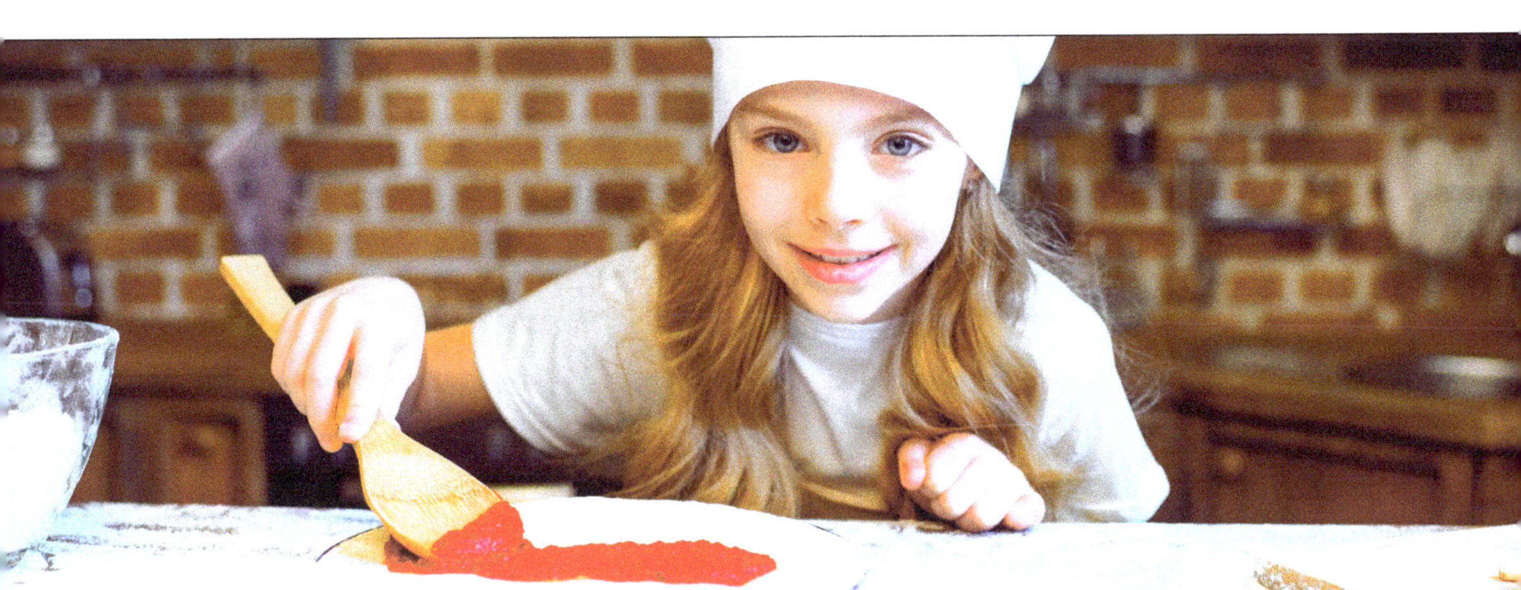

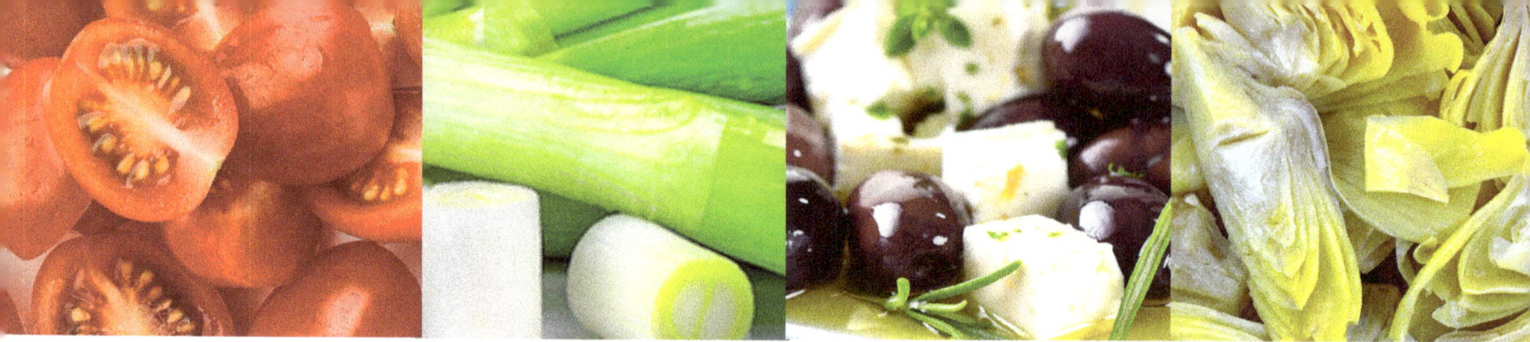

make your greek pizzas!

drizzle+spread+pinch+press

Drizzle your sheet pan with a small amount of olive oil and coat the pan with your hands or with a pastry brush. Wipe hands clean of oil on a damp towel. Pinch dough into small balls (between the sizes of a golf ball and a tennis ball) and press them with your palms to flatten them into any fun shape you want, no thicker than ½ an inch. Kids love how the dough feels! Arrange flattened pizza discs on the oiled sheet pan.

spread+top+bake+eat!

Spread a small amount of pizza sauce on each pizza crust in any fun way you like. We suggest using the back of a metal spoon and to make an even layer, stopping just before the edges of the crust. Top each pizza with an even layer of chopped veggies, **spinach, 1 teaspoon of oregano,** shred and add the **mozzarella** and add the **feta cheese**. Bake 15 to 18 minutes or until cheese is melted and crusts are golden brown!

Mealtime Chatter: How will you top the pizzas the next time you make this dish? Which additional ingredients might you include on your next pizzas?

Banana peppers, or sun-dried tomatoes perhaps?

Time for a Laugh!

How do you fix a broken pizza?

With tomato paste!

What would pizza say if it could talk?

Probably a lot of cheesy things.

Why did the chef open a pizzeria?

Because they KNEADED the dough!

Magical Shakshuka Poached Eggs
+ Pronto Pita Bread
+ Pineapple Orange Spritzers

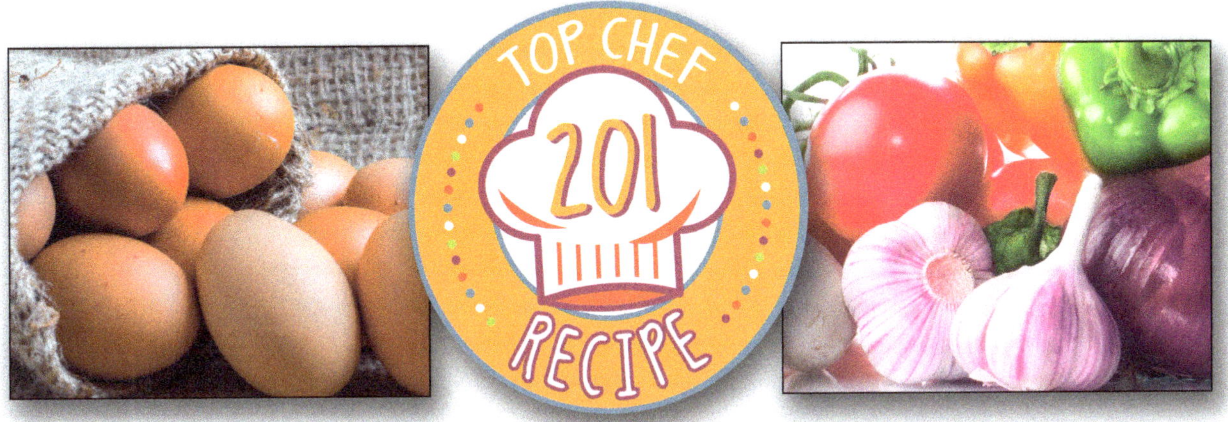

Shakshuka (shahk-SHOO-kah) is a staple dish in northern African and Middle Eastern cuisine, consisting of eggs cooked in a thick, spicy sauce. It's often served as a breakfast dish in Western cuisine because of the use of eggs but traditionally it's eaten for supper! You get to choose...serve for breakfast or dinner?

magical shakshuka poached eggs

ingredients

½ bunch green onions
1 green or red bell pepper
4 large tomatoes
2 garlic cloves
4 T olive oil
2 tsp paprika
½ tsp cumin
1 T tomato paste
2 tsp honey or sugar
1 tsp salt
pinch pepper
6 eggs
½ C feta cheese (optional)
handful fresh parsley

chop+soften

Have your kids chop ½ **bunch green onions, 1 bell pepper,** and **4 tomatoes** into bite-sized pieces and mince **2 garlic cloves** into tiny pieces. Place each vegetable in its own small bowl and set aside. Heat **4 tablespoons of olive oil** in a skillet on your stovetop over medium heat and add the garlic and green onions along with **2 teaspoons of paprika** and ½ **a teaspoon of cumin**. Stir until the onion is soft, about 3 minutes.

add+simmer

To the skillet add your chopped bell pepper and cook until soft, about 3 minutes. Add the chopped tomatoes, **1 tablespoon of tomato paste, 2 teaspoons of sugar or honey, 1 teaspoon of salt,** and **a pinch of pepper**. Stir well and simmer for 10 minutes or until the sauce thickens.

crack+slip+poach

One by one crack **6 eggs** into a small bowl and slip each into the tomato sauce in the skillet before cracking the next egg. Cover the skillet with a lid and poach the eggs until the whites are firm and the yolks have thickened but are not too hard, about 5 minutes.

crumble+sprinkle

Crumble ½ **a cup of feta cheese** and sprinkle some torn **parsley leaves** on top. If the tomato sauce is too dry, add a few tablespoons of water. Serve with *Pronto Pita Bread* and *Pineapple Orange Spritzers*—YUM!

pronto pita bread

ingredients

- 1¼ C all-purpose flour
- 1 tsp active dry yeast
- ½ tsp sugar
- ½ tsp salt
- ½ C warm water
- 2 tsp olive oil

measure+mix

In a large mixing bowl, combine 1¼ **cups of flour, 1 teaspoon of yeast,** ½ **a teaspoon of sugar,** and ½ **a teaspoon of salt**. Slowly add in ½ **a cup of warm water** and **2 teaspoon of olive oil**. Encourage kids to mix with clean hands by pushing the dough with their palms and turning, kneading about 50 times. Don't worry—the dough should be sticky!

cover+rest

Turn the dough out on a floured surface and cover with a dishtowel. Let the dough rest for at least 10 minutes and up to 2 hours.

preheat+divide+shape

Preheat a skillet on your stovetop over medium-high heat. Divide your dough into 8 to 12 pieces, depending how large you like your pita bread. Have your kids shape each piece of dough into a ball and then flatten each ball into a circle.

cook+flip

Carefully cook the dough on your hot skillet, about 1 minute per side, flipping to cook each side. Serve warm.

pineapple orange spritzers

ingredients

1 to 2 oranges
1 C pineapple juice
2 C sparkling water
2 C ice

peel+pour

Peel the skin of **1 to 2 oranges** and add fruit into a regular blender or pitcher (if using an immersion blender). Discard the peels. Pour in **1 cup of pineapple juice.**

blend+stir

Blend the oranges and pineapple juice together until smooth. Pour **2 cups of sparkling water** over the top and mix well with a large spoon. Add **2 cups of ice**, serve, and ENJOY!

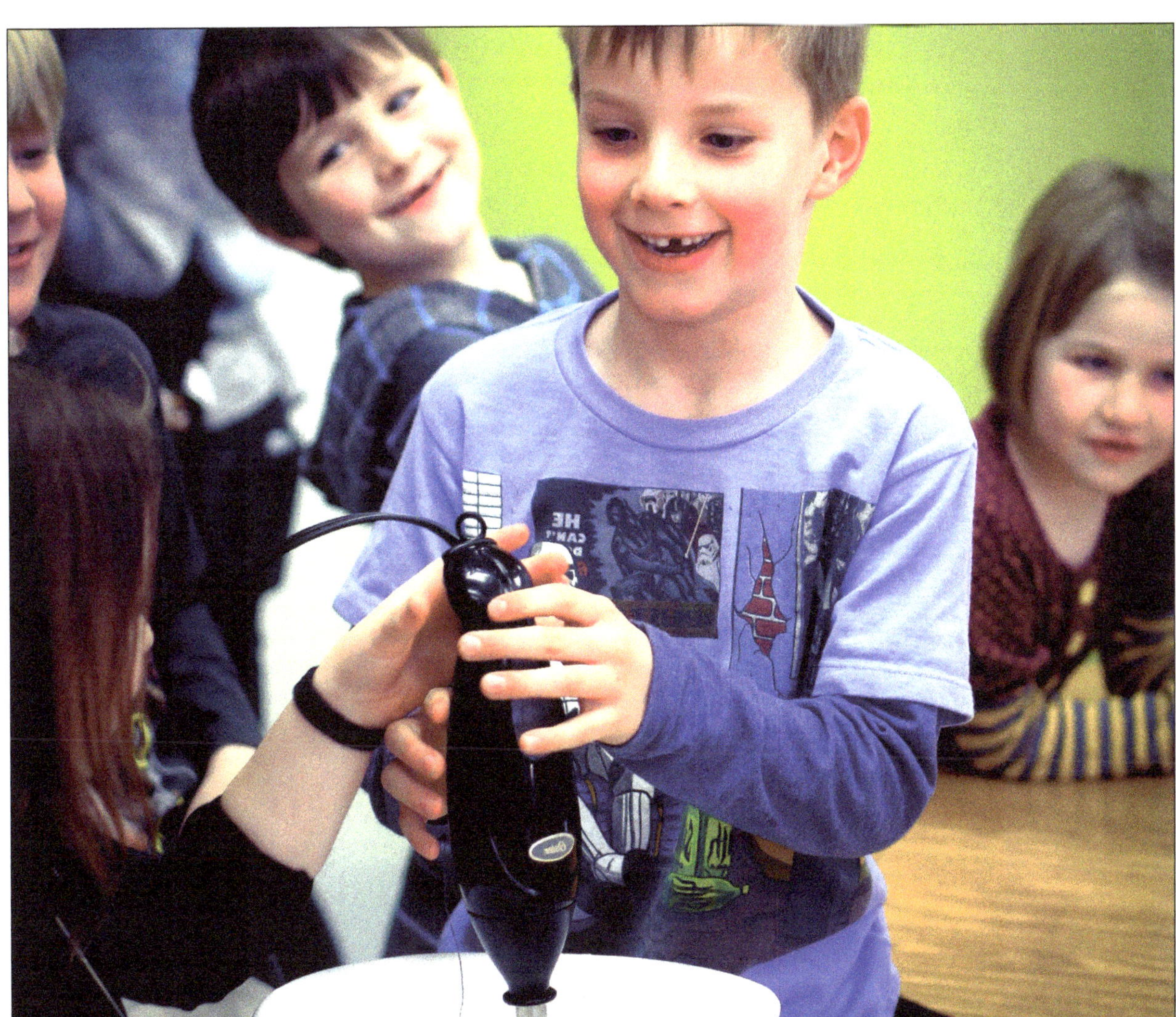

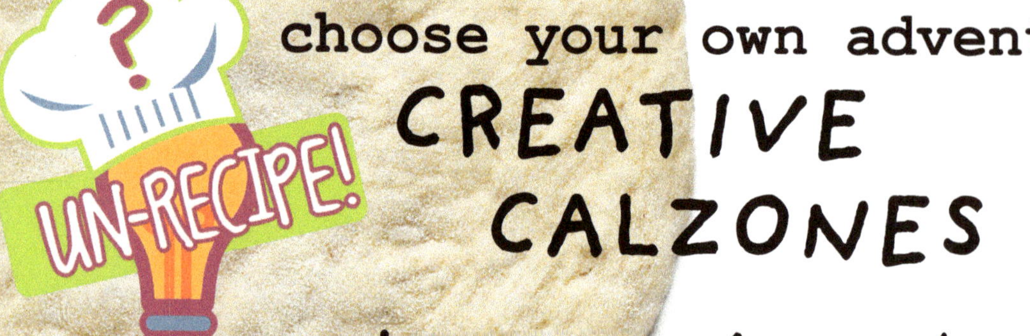

choose your own adventure!

CREATIVE CALZONES

make your pizza dough!

Start by mixing **4 cups of flour, 1 teaspoon of baking powder, and 1 teaspoon of salt.** Stir in **2 cups of yogurt** and mix until a large ball forms. Add flour by the tablespoon if the dough is too sticky to handle. Turn dough out onto a floured surface, kneading the dough for about 5 minutes until the dough feels smooth and elastic. Roll dough into a ball, place in the bottom of an oiled bowl, and cover with a damp dish towel. Let dough rest while you prepare your add-ins.

sweet calzones:

choose 1 base:

ricotta cheese
cream cheese
fruit jam
seed or nut butter

chose 2+ add-ins (or create your own!):

chopped apples
applesauce
raisins
chocolate chips
berries
sugar
cinnamon

savory calzones:

choose 1 sauce:

tomato sauce
green pesto
sun-dried tomato pesto
alfredo sauce

chose 2+ add-ins (or create your own!):

mozzarella cheese
ricotta cheese
fresh spinach
chopped bell pepper
chopped zucchini
chopped mushrooms
chopped tomatoes
garlic powder
salt + pepper

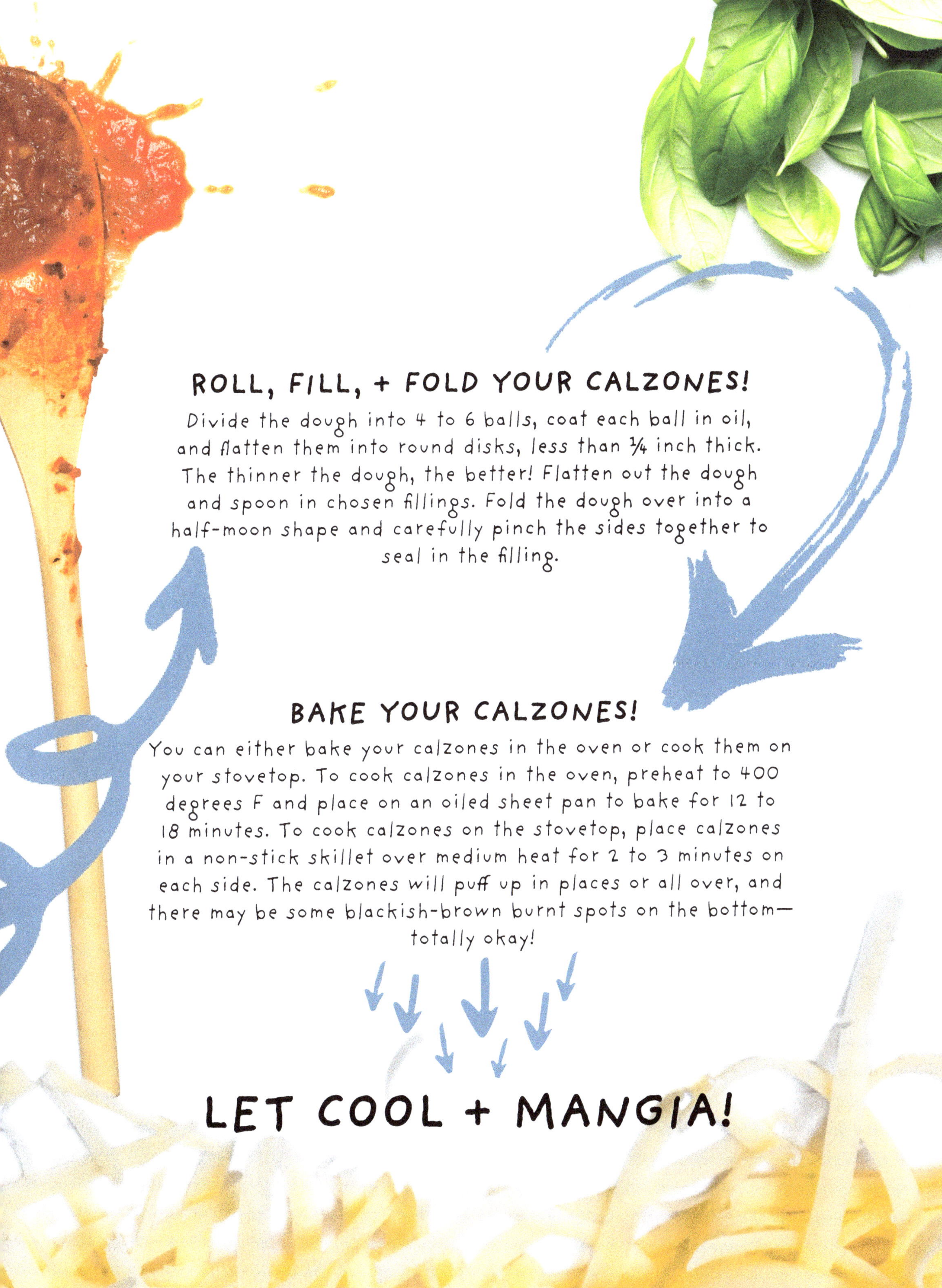

ROLL, FILL, + FOLD YOUR CALZONES!

Divide the dough into 4 to 6 balls, coat each ball in oil, and flatten them into round disks, less than ¼ inch thick. The thinner the dough, the better! Flatten out the dough and spoon in chosen fillings. Fold the dough over into a half-moon shape and carefully pinch the sides together to seal in the filling.

BAKE YOUR CALZONES!

You can either bake your calzones in the oven or cook them on your stovetop. To cook calzones in the oven, preheat to 400 degrees F and place on an oiled sheet pan to bake for 12 to 18 minutes. To cook calzones on the stovetop, place calzones in a non-stick skillet over medium heat for 2 to 3 minutes on each side. The calzones will puff up in places or all over, and there may be some blackish-brown burnt spots on the bottom—totally okay!

LET COOL + MANGIA!

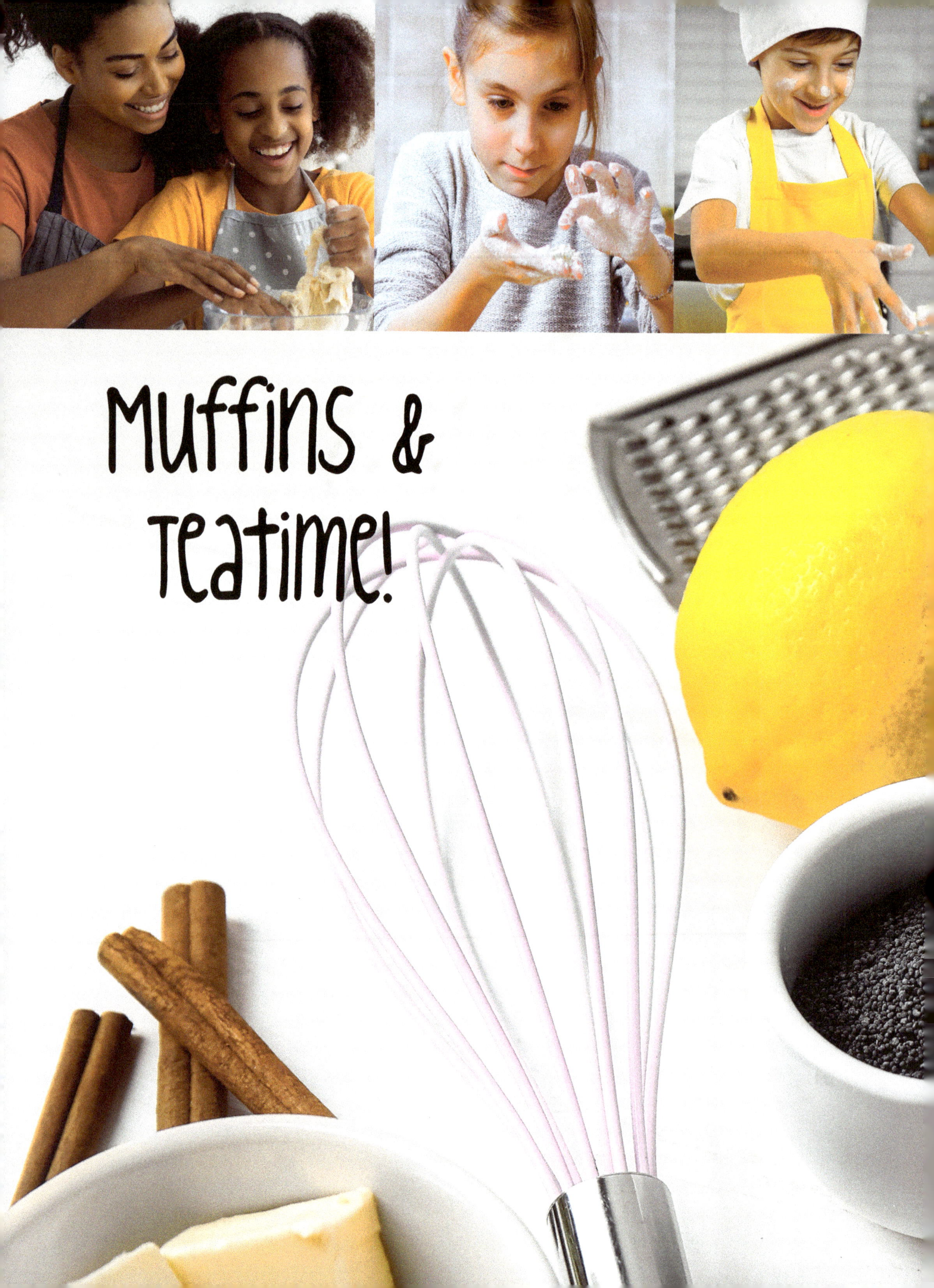

Muffins & Teatime!

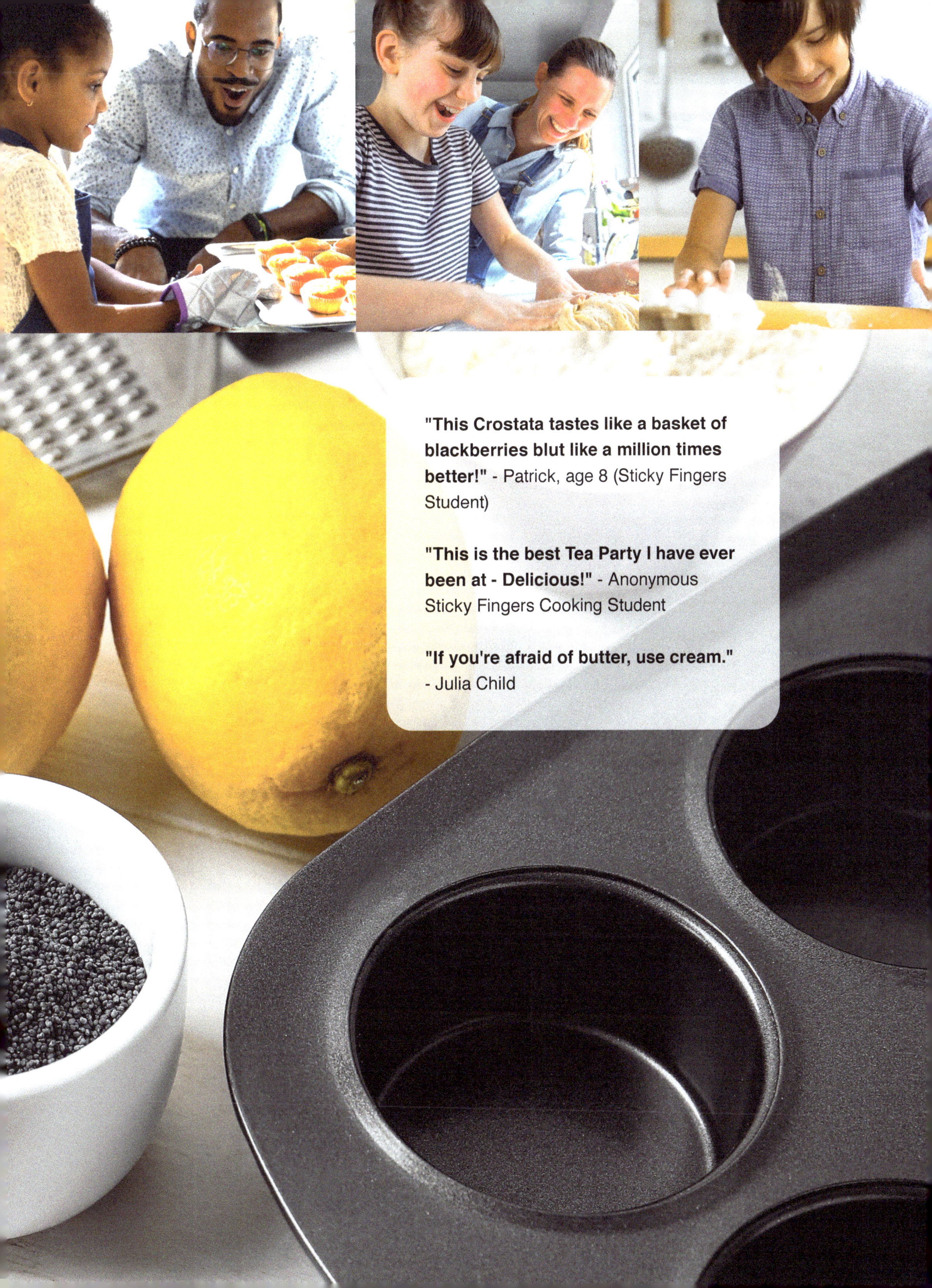

"This Crostata tastes like a basket of blackberries blut like a million times better!" - Patrick, age 8 (Sticky Fingers Student)

"This is the best Tea Party I have ever been at - Delicious!" - Anonymous Sticky Fingers Cooking Student

"If you're afraid of butter, use cream." - Julia Child

Beautifully Basic Scones

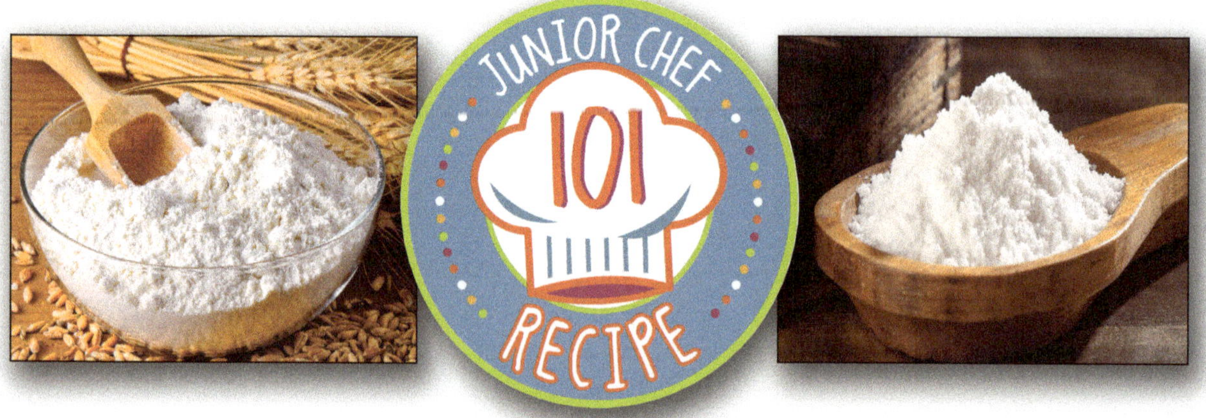

beautifully basic scones

ingredients

2 C all-purpose flour + more if needed
3½ tsp baking powder
2 T + 1 tsp sugar (+ more to sprinkle)
1 tsp salt
1½ C whipping cream (sub 1 can full-fat coconut milk)

preheat+measure+combine+mix

Preheat oven to 400 degrees F. First, make your scone dough! In a large mixing bowl, add **2 cups of flour, 3½ teaspoons of baking powder, 2 tablespoons and 1 teaspoon of sugar,** and **1 teaspoon of salt** and mix. Add **1½ cups of whipping cream**. Mix with a spoon until all bits of flour disappear, but don't over-mix! If dough is too sticky add up to ¼ cup of flour. Set aside dough.

choose+chop+mix

Now for the really fun part! Choose your creative **add-in ingredients** making your scones either sweet or savory: chopped fruit, herbs, chocolate chips, cheese, etc. in any combination you like. Chop and mix together add-in ingredients to the dough.

divide+fold+flatten

Divide the dough into 12 pieces. Sprinkle some flour onto a clean, flat surface (like a cutting board or countertop). Then flatten the scones a bit with your hands until they are no more than an inch thick.

brush+bake

Brush each scone with whipping cream and sprinkle with sugar. Arrange scones on a parchment-lined baking sheet, bake for about 20 to 25 minutes or until golden brown on top!

Have fun selecting sweet or savory add-in ingredients to your scones!

creative savory add-ins:

cheddar/gouda/Parmesan cheese
bell peppers or jalapeños
dried herbs
chives
bacon (precooked)
diced ham
olives

creative sweet scone add-ins:

dried, fresh, or frozen (thawed) fruit
chocolate chips
shredded coconut
cinnamon
lemon or orange zest
candied ginger

Mealtime Chatter: How do you like the flavors and textures of your creative add-ins? What will you do differently the next time you make scones?

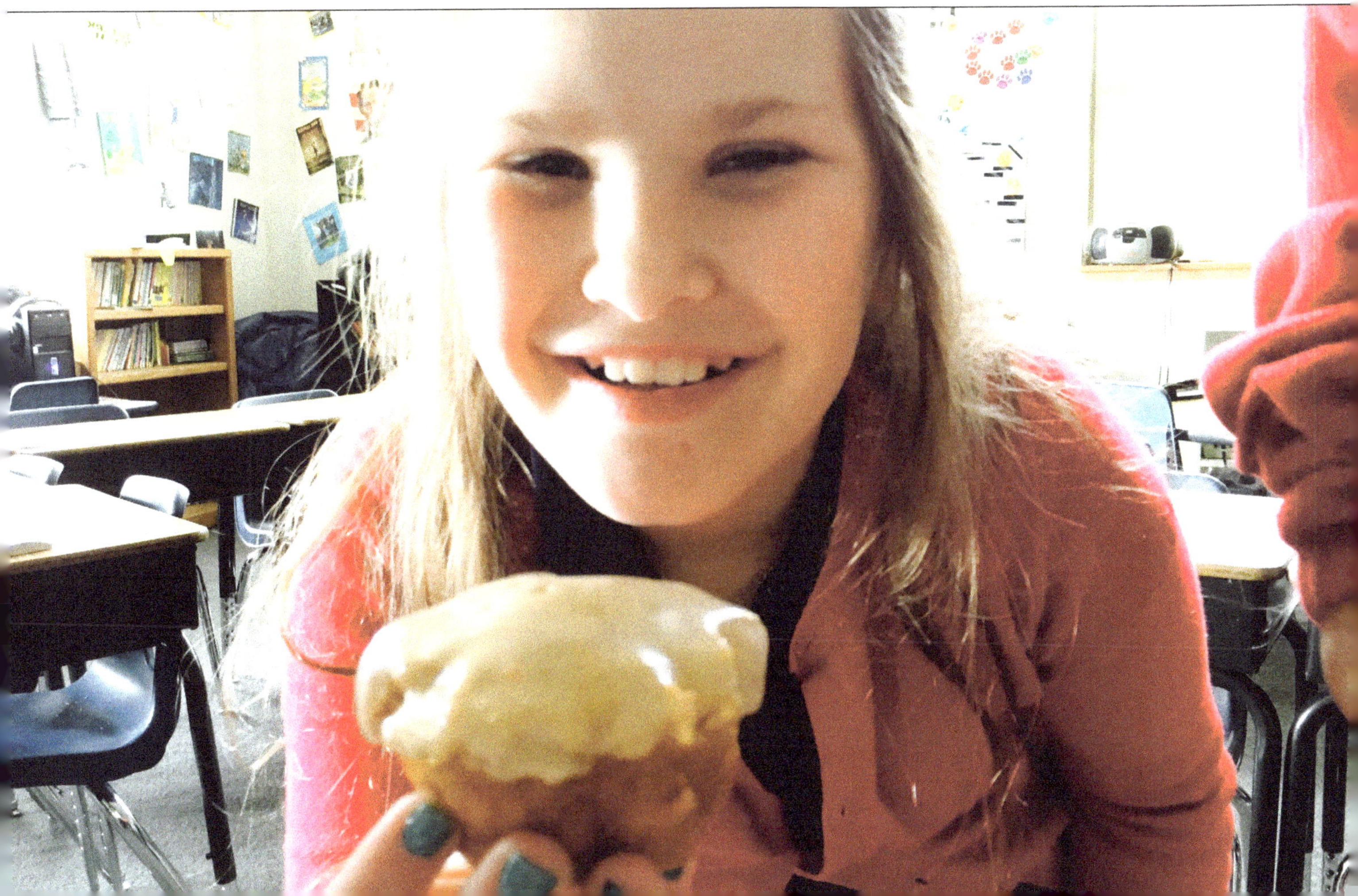

Blackberry Lime Corn Love Muffins

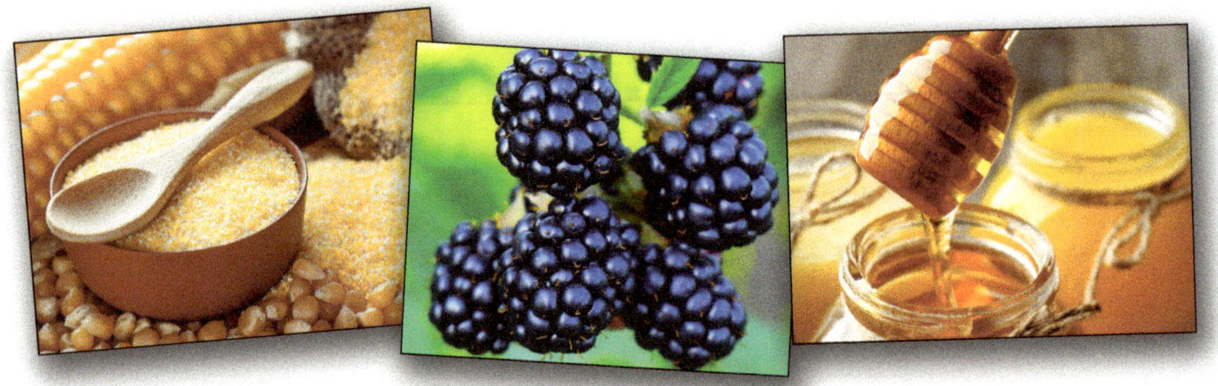

blackberry lime corn love muffins

ingredients

¾ C all-purpose flour
1 ½ tsp baking powder
½ C yellow cornmeal
½ C milk
⅓ C honey
¼ C unsalted butter
½ C fresh or frozen (thawed) blackberries
2 eggs (sub ¼ cup silken tofu)
1 lime

mix+measure

Preheat oven to 375 degrees F. Have kids measure and add ¾ **cup of flour, 1½ teaspoons of baking powder,** and ½ **cup of cornmeal** to a medium bowl. Mix and set aside.

wet+measure

In a medium bowl, have your kids measure out ½ **cup of milk,** ⅓ **cup of honey,** ¼ **cup of butter** and ½ **cup of blackberries**. Mix together and set aside.

crack+squeeze

Crack **2 eggs** over a small bowl and separate the yolks from the whites and then add yolks to the wet bowl. Cut **1 lime** in half and squeeze the juice into the wet ingredients bowl.

CUPCAKES/MUFFINS: Try using an ice cream scoop to evenly measure cupcake or muffin batter into the tin wells!

mix

Mix the wet and dry ingredients together and stir just enough to combine. The batter should look beautiful and purple! Be cautious to not overmix.

pour+bake

Pour the lined wells of a muffin pan ½ full of batter and bake for 20 to 30 minutes or until golden brown, or until a toothpick comes out clean when poked through the center of a muffin.

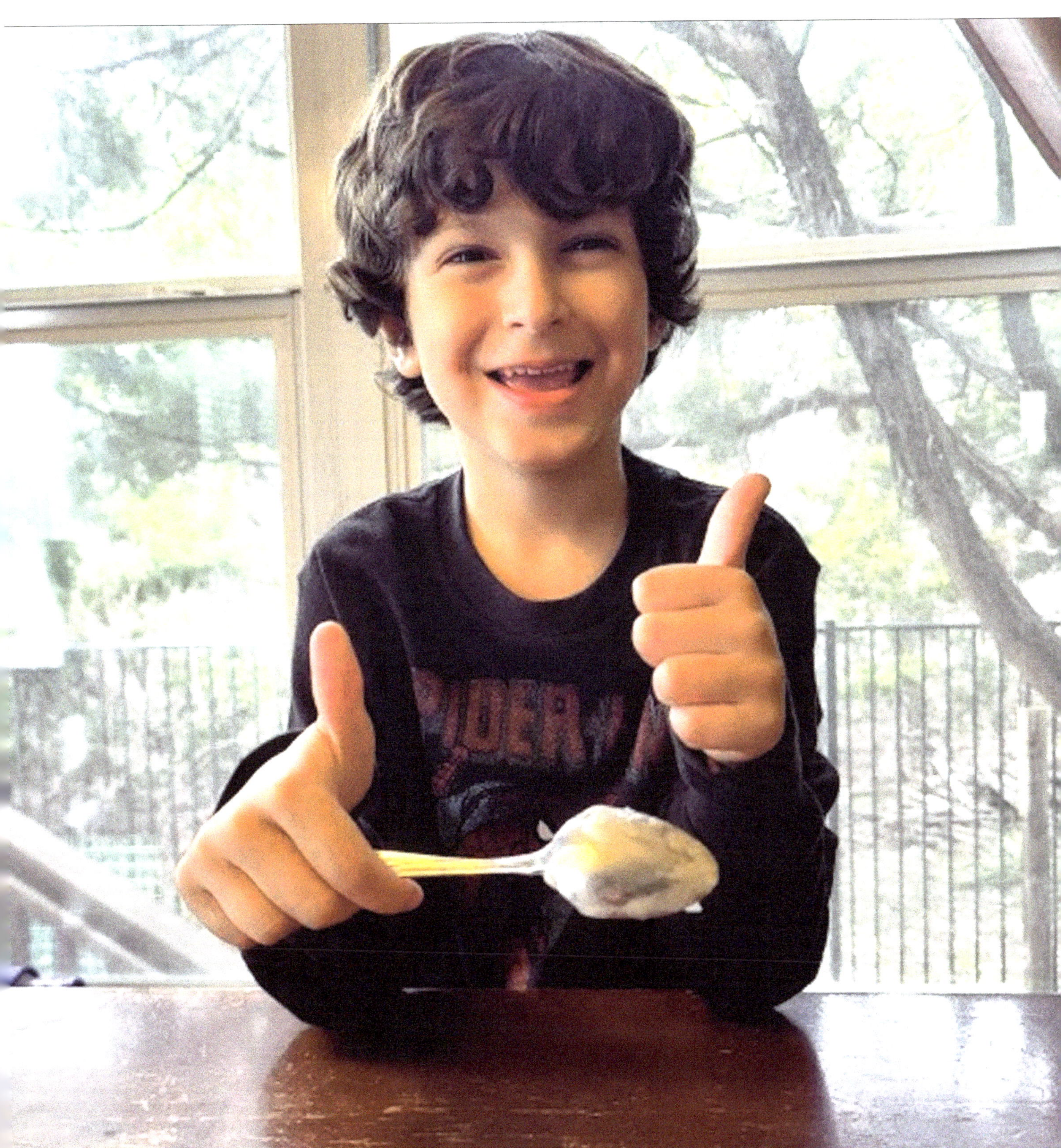

Mandarin Orange Muffins

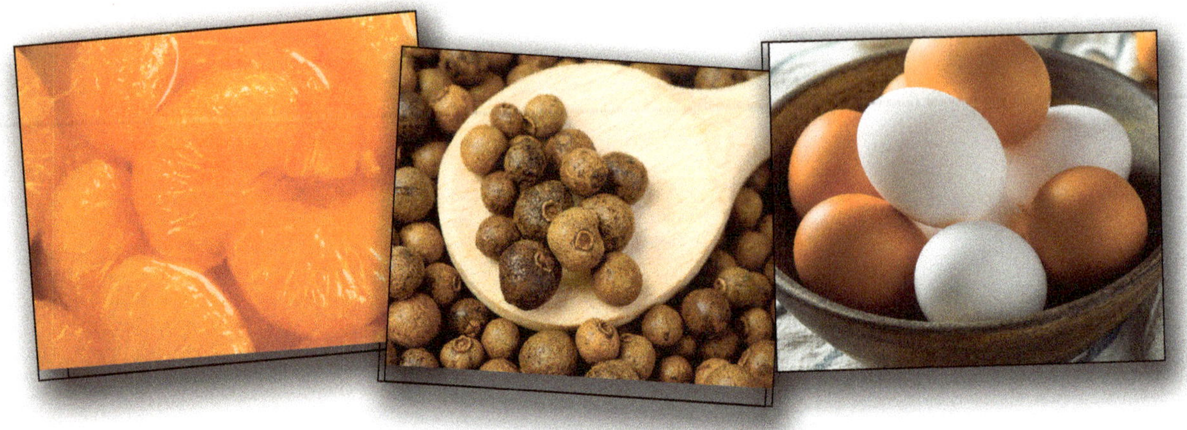

mandarin orange muffins

ingredients

1½ C all-purpose flour
1¾ tsp baking powder
½ tsp salt
¼ tsp allspice
¼ tsp nutmeg
½ C sugar
⅓ C unsalted butter
1 egg
1 to 2 fresh oranges (juice)
2 cans Mandarin oranges
pinch sugar

mix+measure

Preheat your oven to 350 degrees F. Have kids mix **1½ cups of flour, 1¾ teaspoons of baking powder, ½ teaspoon of salt, ¼ teaspoon of allspice, ¼ teaspoon of nutmeg** and ½ **cup of sugar**.

cut+crumble

Have your kids soften ⅓ **cup of butter** and cut into the dry ingredients until the mixture crumbles into pea-sized pieces.

beat+squeeze

Have your kids beat **1 egg** and set aside. Take turns squeezing juice from **1 or 2 oranges** until you have ¼ **cup of orange juice**. Add the orange juice and egg to the dry ingredients mix and incorporate until just moistened.

fold+bake

Have your kids carefully drain **1 can of Mandarin Oranges** and fold into the batter. Fill a paper lined muffin pan ¾ full of batter, then top muffins with one Mandarin slice and a pinch of sugar. Enjoy snacking on the rest of the mandarin oranges as the muffins bake. Bake for 12 to 18 minutes, or until baked through. Let cool and ENJOY!

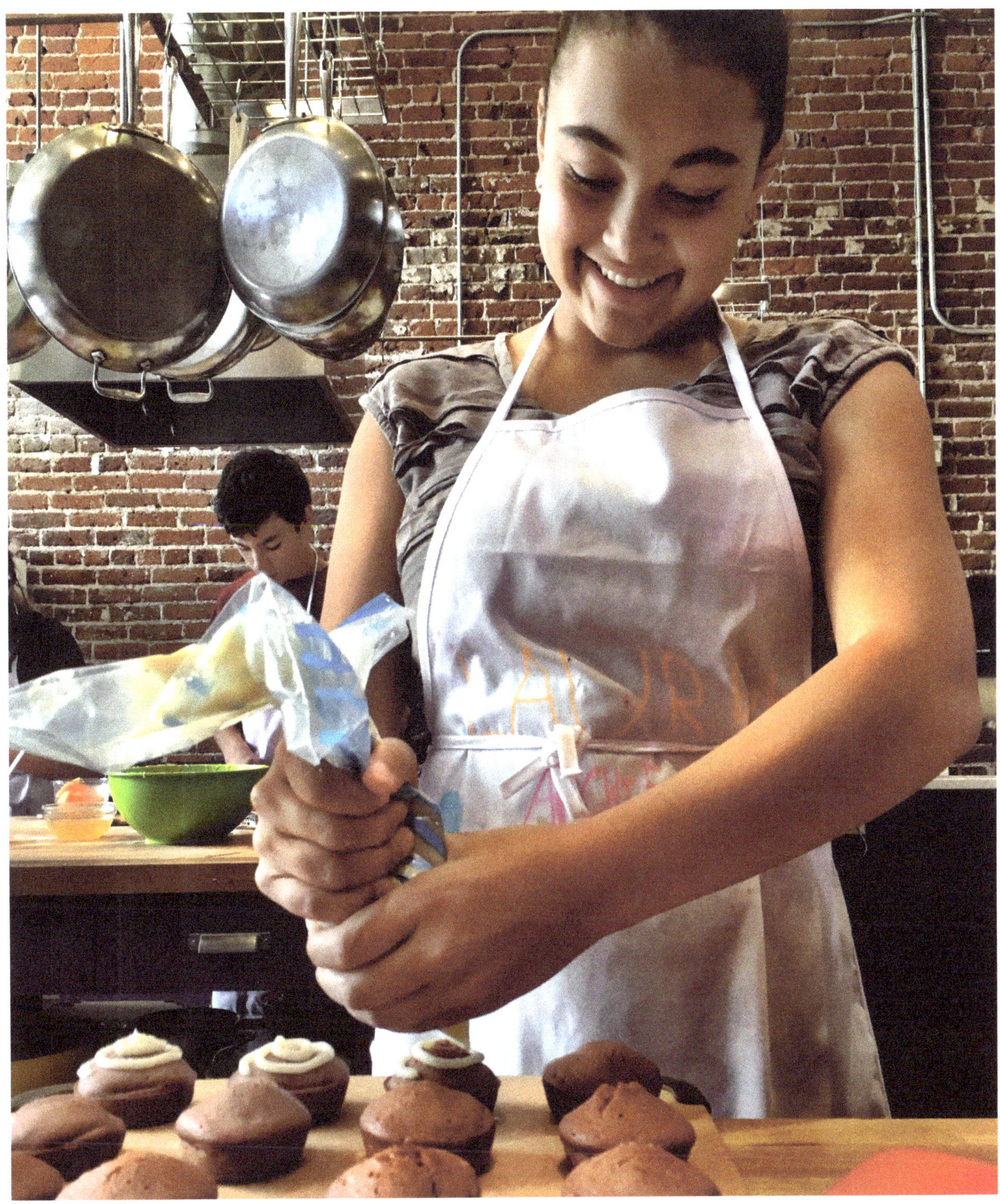

Oatmeal Cookie Muffins

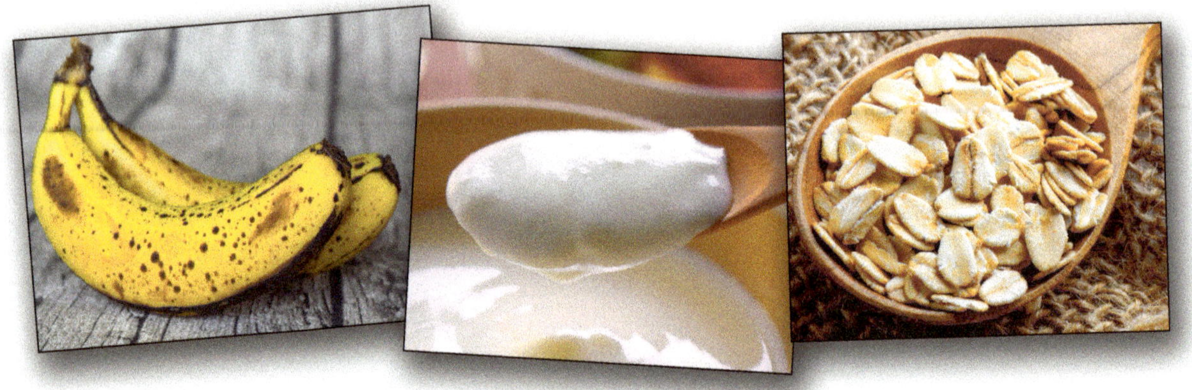

oatmeal cookie muffins

ingredients

½ C raisins
2 ripe bananas
1 C old-fashioned oats
1 C all-purpose flour
½ C brown sugar
2 tsp baking powder
½ tsp baking soda
1 tsp cinnamon
¾ C plain whole-milk yogurt
¾ C milk
2 large eggs
1 tsp vanilla extract
¼ C chocolate chips
2 T unsalted butter (sub vegetable oil)

preheat+plump+blend

Preheat your oven to 350 degrees F. Plump up ½ **cup of raisins** by heating some water in a small saucepan on your stovetop and adding the raisins for a few minutes until soft. Drain the water. Mash **2 bananas** until they form a paste. Then blend the bananas and softened raisins into a thick paste with an immersion blender/regular blender/food processor.

measure+mix

Have kids measure and mix together the dry ingredients in a large bowl: **1 cup of oats, 1 cup of flour, ½ cup of brown sugar, 2 teaspoons of baking powder, ½ teaspoon of baking soda,** and **1 teaspoon of cinnamon**. Measure and mix together the wet ingredients in a medium bowl: **¾ cup of yogurt, ¾ cup of milk, 2 eggs,** and **1 teaspoon of vanilla extract**.

whisk+fold+stir

Whisk the wet ingredients into the dry until just combined and then fold in the banana/raisin mixture, along with ¼ **cup of chocolate chips**. Finally, soften **2 tablespoons of butter or oil** and stir into the batter.

bake+serve

Fill the lined wells of a muffin pan ½ full of batter. Bake for 10 to 15 minutes, or until a toothpick inserted in the center of a muffin comes out clean.

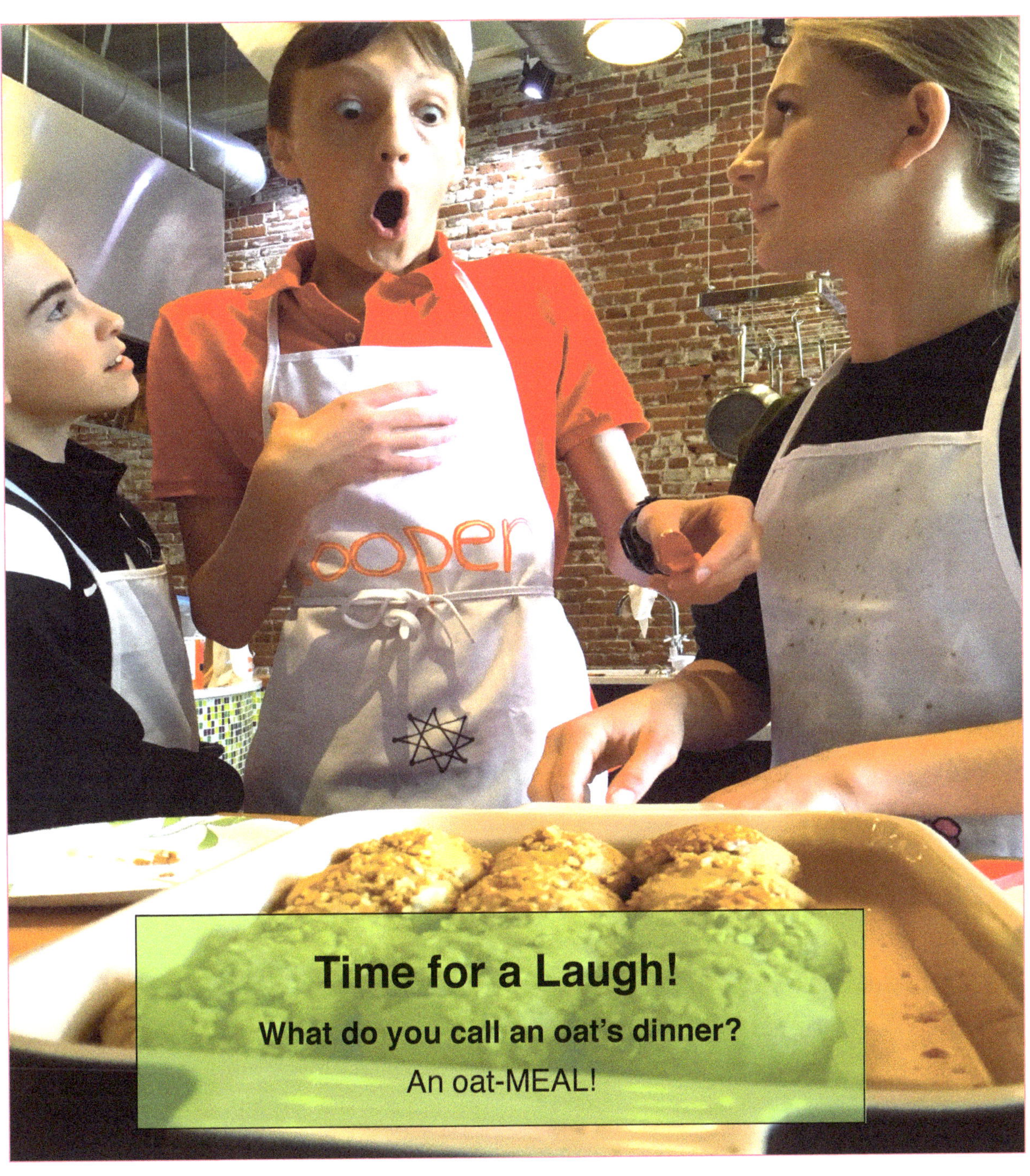

Time for a Laugh!

What do you call an oat's dinner?

An oat-MEAL!

Banana Split Cherry Muffins

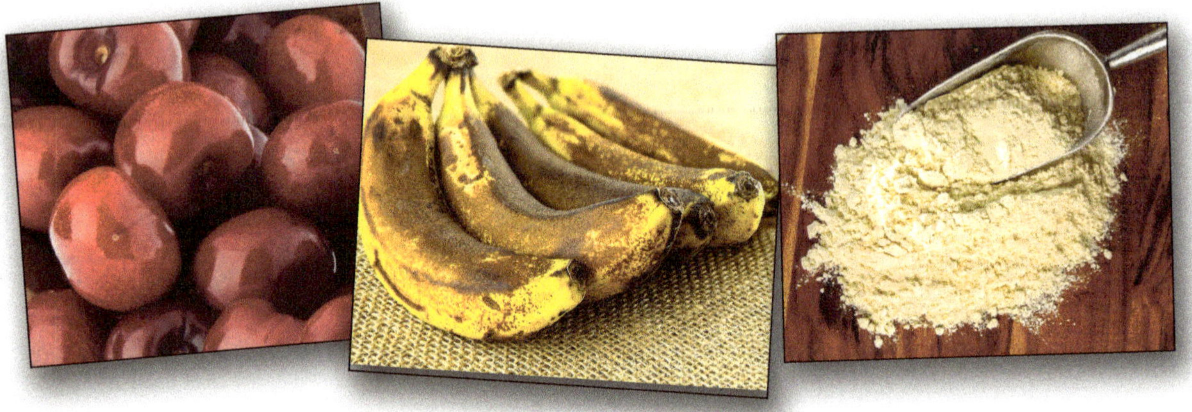

banana split cherry muffins

ingredients

3 very ripe bananas
½ C frozen (thawed) cherries
1 orange (zest)
¾ C white or brown sugar
2 extra-large eggs
½ C vegetable oil
½ C sour cream
1 tsp vanilla extract
2 C all-purpose flour
1 tsp baking soda
½ tsp kosher salt
handful chocolate chips (optional)
oil or butter (for greasing pan)

preheat+chop+zest

Preheat your oven to 350 degrees F. Have your kids chop up **3 bananas** and ½ **cup of cherries** into small pieces for the muffin batter. Zest **1 orange**—be careful to only grate the orange part and stop grating when you see the white pith!

measure+whisk

Measure ¾ **cup of sugar** and add to the chopped bananas. Whisk well until combined.

crack+combine

Invite your kids to crack **2 eggs** into the bowl with the sugar and bananas. Then add ½ **cup of vegetable oil,** ½ **cup of sour cream, 1 teaspoon of vanilla extract,** and the orange zest. Mix well until smooth.

measure+mix

Time for the dry ingredients! In a new bowl, measure **2 cups of flour, 1 teaspoon of baking soda,** and ½ **teaspoon of salt**. Whisk the dry ingredients and the wet ingredients together until combined. If using **handful of chocolate chips**, stir them in now.

fill+bake

Line a muffin pan with paper liners or grease with **oil or butter**. Fill each well ⅔ full with batter. Bake 20 to 25 minutes, or until a toothpick inserted in the center of a muffin comes out clean. Let cool completely.

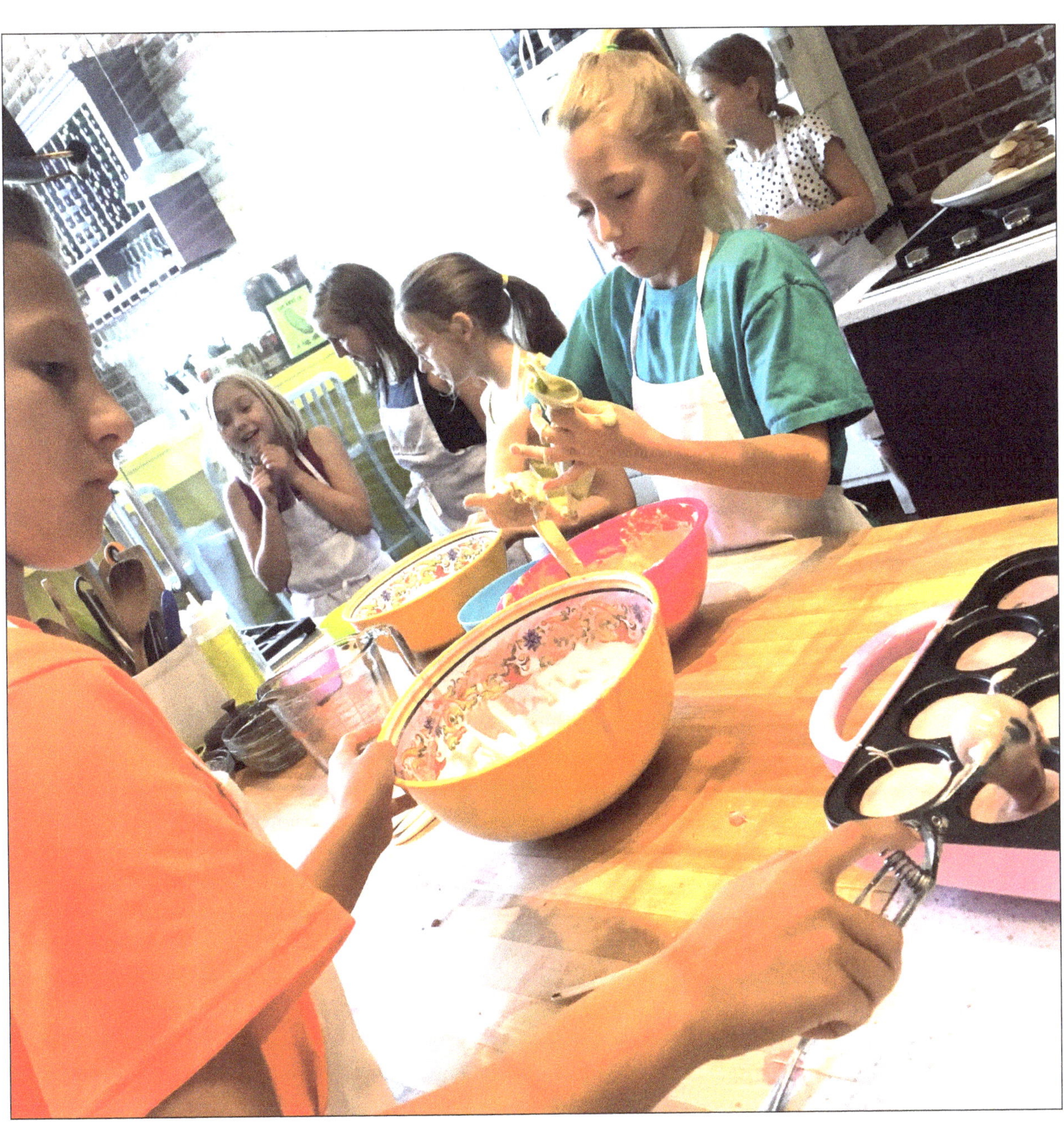

Sticky Icky Toffee Date Muffins
+ Quick Salted Caramel

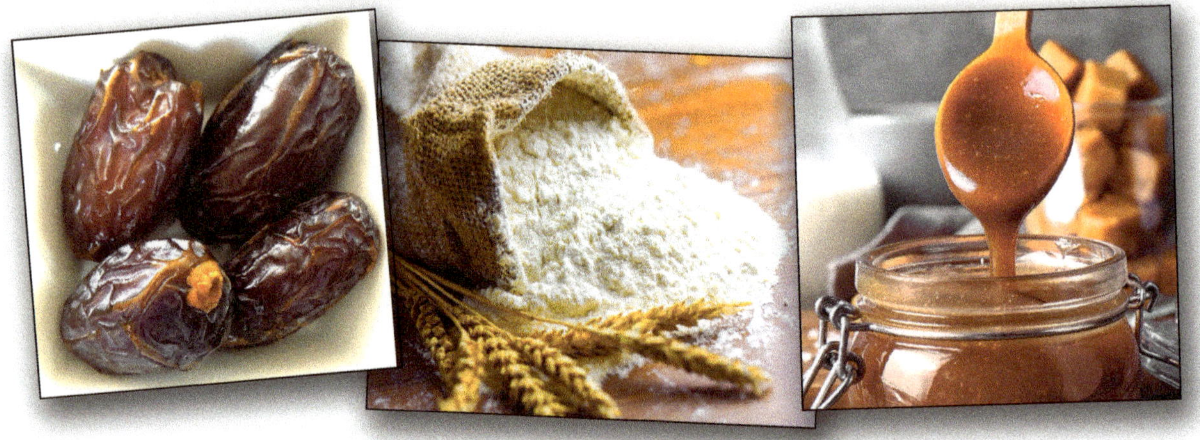

sticky icky toffee date muffins

ingredients

8 to 10 pitted dates
1 T fresh lemon juice
½ C raisins
1½ C all-purpose flour
1½ tsp pumpkin pie spice
1 tsp baking soda
1¾ sticks unsalted butter
¾ C (packed) light brown sugar
2 eggs
½ tsp vanilla extract

chop+squeeze+simmer

Have your kids chop up **8 to 10 dates** and squeeze **1 tablespoon of lemon juice**. Bring chopped dates, lemon juice, and ¾ cup water to a boil in a small saucepan on your stovetop. Reduce heat and simmer gently until the chopped dates soften and start to fall apart, about 3 to 6 minutes. Add ½ **cup of raisins** to the saucepan, remove from heat, and set aside to cool completely.

preheat+measure+stir

While the date mixture cools, preheat your oven to 325 degrees F. In a medium bowl, measure and combine your dry ingredients: **1½ cups of flour, 1½ teaspoons of pumpkin pie spice, ¾ teaspoon of salt,** and **1 teaspoon of baking soda**.

combine+cream

In a large mixing bowl, cream **1¾ sticks of butter** and ¾ **cup of light brown sugar** together with a hand mixer or blender until light and fluffy, about 3 to 5 minutes.

crack+purée+whisk

Encourage kids to crack **2 eggs** into the butter mixture, mixing well after each addition and scraping down the sides of the bowl as needed. Measure and mix ½ **teaspoon of vanilla extract** into the cooled date mixture and purée until smooth. For the final step, whisk the dry ingredients into the wet ingredients until combined.

fill+bake

Fill the lined wells of a muffin pan ½ full of batter and bake for 15 to 20 minutes or until a toothpick inserted into the center comes out mostly clean with just a few crumbs stuck to it.

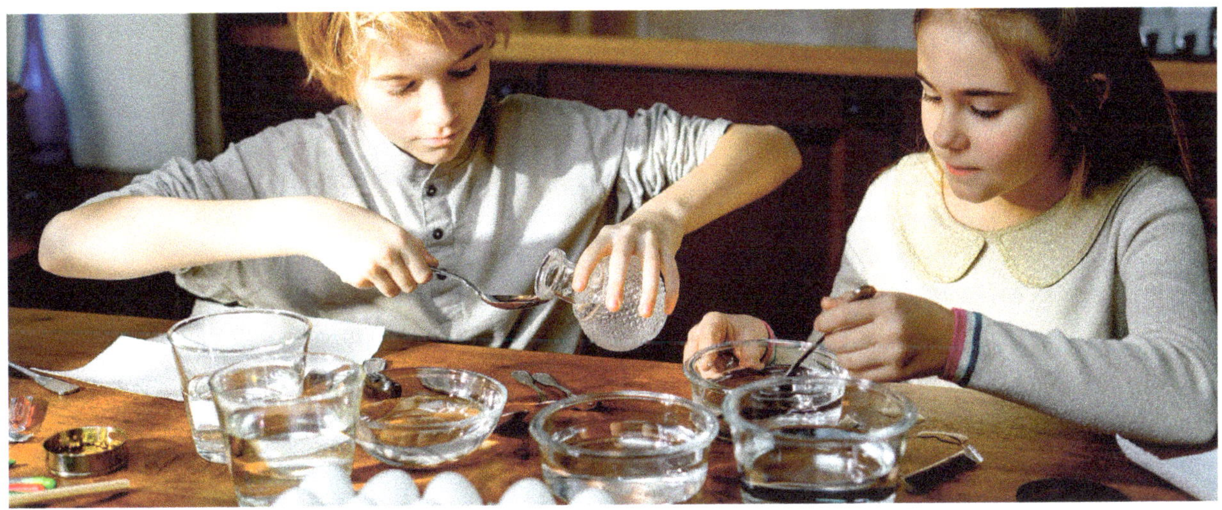

quick salted caramel

ingredients

¼ C agave nectar or honey
¼ C light brown sugar
⅛ tsp salt
1 T unsalted butter

simmer+whisk

In a small saucepan on your stovetop, combine ¼ **cup of agave nectar or honey,** ¼ **cup of light brown sugar,** and ⅛ **teaspoon of salt** and bring to a simmer over medium heat, whisking to dissolve the sugar. Once the sugar dissolves and bubbles, remove from heat and swirl in **1 tablespoon of butter**.

French Apple Turnovers
+ Citron Crème Glacée

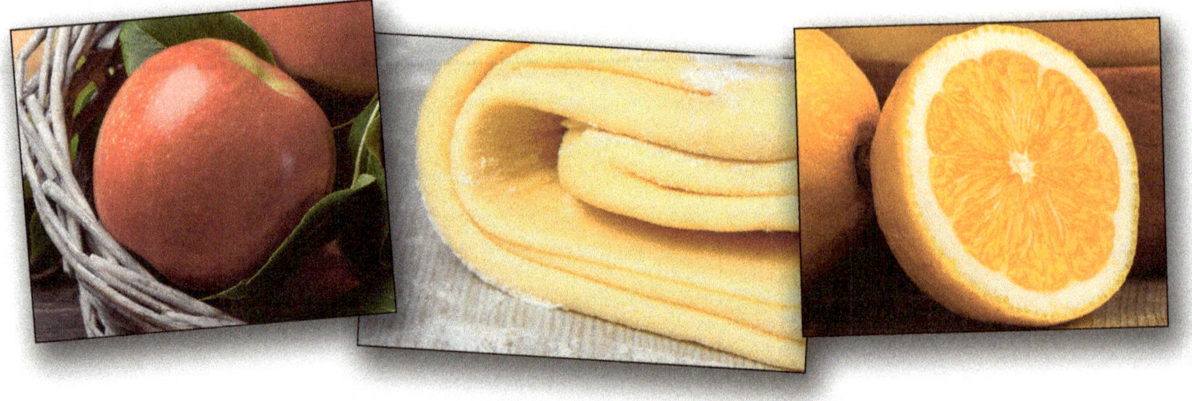

french apple turnovers

ingredients

10 oz frozen (thawed) puff pastry
1 lemon (zest)
1 large apple
¼ cup sugar
2 tsp cornstarch
½ tsp salt
all-purpose flour (for dusting)
round cookie cutter or the lid of a mason jar

thaw+preheat+zest+chop

Thaw **10 ounces of frozen puff pastry** in fridge overnight or for at least 6 hours. Preheat oven to 350 degrees F. Wash and zest **1 lemon**. Chop **1 apple** into tiny pieces and set aside.

measure+mix+add

In a large mixing bowl, have kids measure and mix together **¼ cup of sugar, 2 teaspoons of cornstarch, ½ teaspoon of salt**, and lemon zest. Add chopped apples and mix to coat them.

roll out+spoon+seal+bake

Sprinkle **some flour** on a clean, flat surface. Onto the surface, roll out thawed puff pastry so that it is even and flat. Using a round cookie cutter or the lid of a mason jar, invite kids to punch circles of the dough. Or, for rectangular-shaped turnovers, cut puff pastry into equal rectangles. Spoon 2 teaspoons of apple filling mixture into the center of each puff pastry shape. Fold over and seal the edges. Place turnovers in muffin pan and bake for 10 to 15 minutes, or until turnovers are golden brown and juices are bubbling. Let cool slightly before serving!

citron crème glacée

ingredients

¼ cup powdered sugar
3 tsp lemon juice
½ tsp vanilla extract
pinch salt

squeeze+whisk

In a small mixing bowl, combine **¼ cup of powdered sugar, 3 teaspoons of lemon juice, ½ teaspoon of vanilla extract**, and **a pinch of salt.** Whisk until a smooth and pourable icing forms.

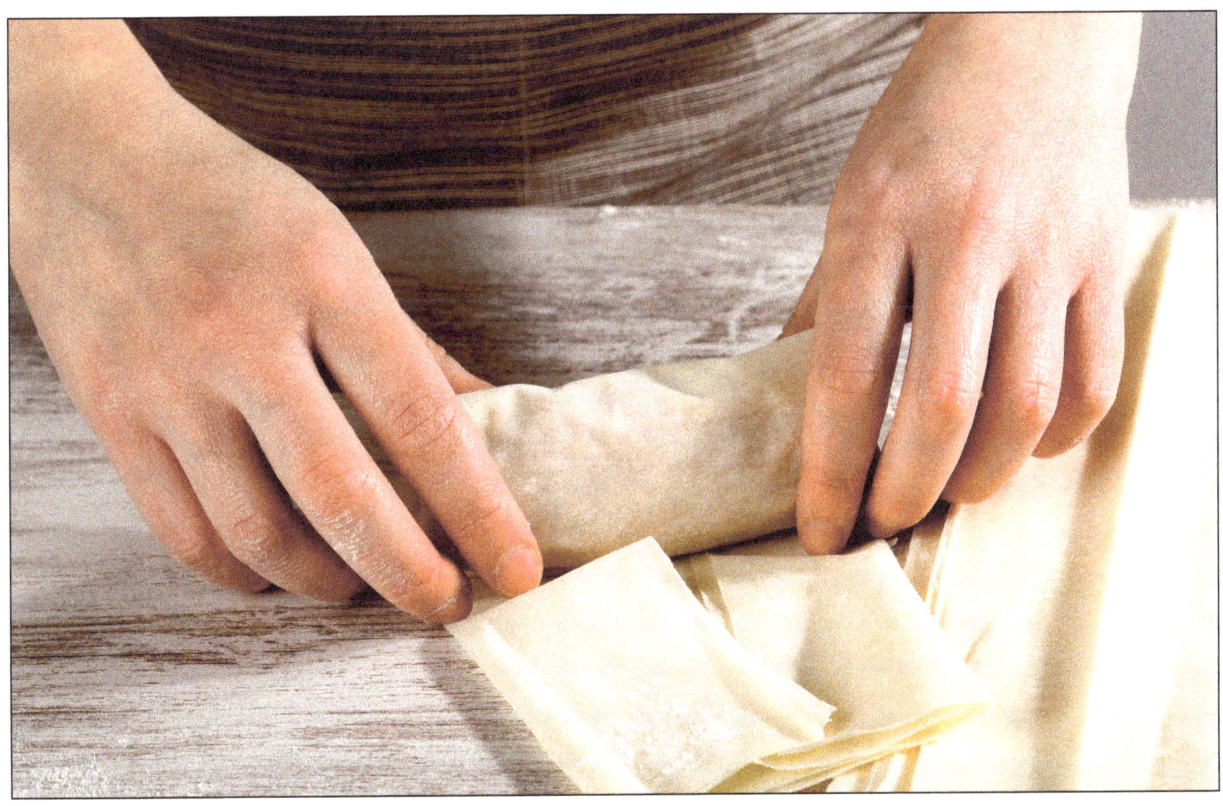

Time for a Laugh!

Why did the pie go to a dentist?

Because he needed a filling!

Italian Bella Fruit Crostada

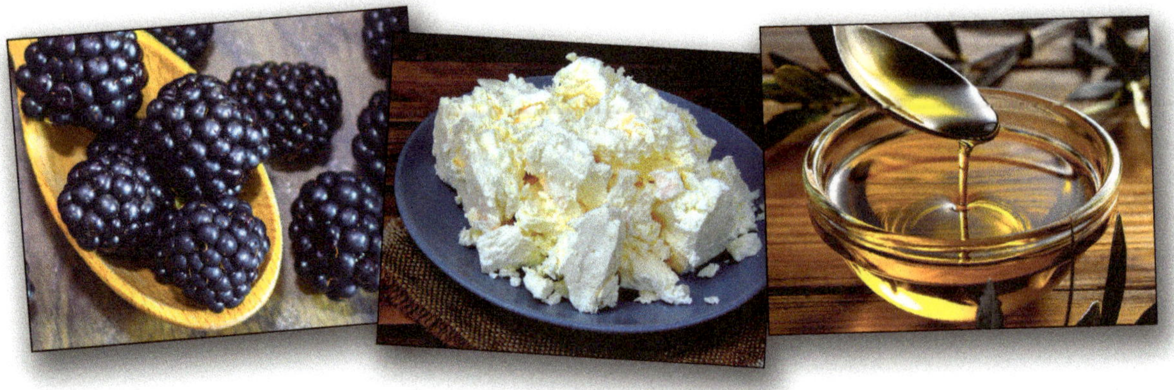

fruit crostata filling

ingredients

1 lemon (zest)
⅓ C sugar (+ more for sprinkling on top)
2 tsp all-purpose flour or cornstarch
½ tsp salt
pinch cinnamon
¾ lb fresh blackberries or plums
4 T ricotta cheese (optional)

zest+measure

Invite your kids to carefully zest the peel of **1 lemon**. In a medium mixing bowl, measure **⅓ cup of sugar, 2 teaspoons of flour or cornstarch, ½ teaspoon of salt, a pinch of cinnamon,** and ½ teaspoon of lemon zest. Mix to combine

squeeze+toss

Add a squeeze of lemon juice to the mixture and then add ¾ **pound of blackberries or plums.** If using plums, slice the plums in half and remove the pits. Chop into small pieces with the skins on (when baked, the skins give a beautiful color and texture). Add **4 heaping tablespoons of ricotta cheese**, if desired. Toss the fruit to coat in the sugar/lemon mixture. Set to the side.

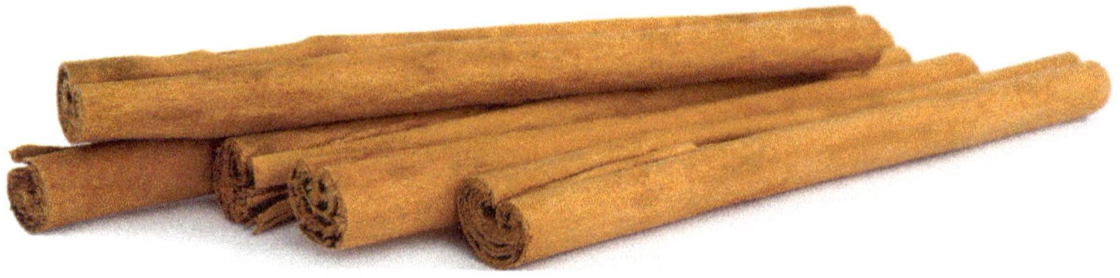

no-roll pie crust dough

ingredients

1⅔ C all-purpose flour
¼ C fine cornmeal
1 tsp sugar
½ tsp baking powder
pinch cinnamon
7 T olive oil
¼ C cold water
1 lemon

preheat+measure+mix

Preheat your oven to 450 degrees F. In a large mixing bowl, measure **1⅔ cups of flour, ¼ cup of cornmeal, ½ teaspoon of salt, 1 teaspoon of sugar, ½ teaspoon of baking powder,** and **a pinch of cinnamon**. Mix the dry ingredients with a fork or whisk.

pour+ball

Have your kids make a well in the center of the dry ingredients and add **7 tablespoons of olive oil, ¼ cup of cold water,** and the zest of **1 lemon** (about ½ teaspoon worth). Mix with a fork or your hands until it makes a ball.

shape+fill

At this point you have a few options for making your rustic, open-face fruit tart crostata:

★ **THE BIG ONE:** Roll out the dough out with a rolling pin or pinch the shape together with your fingers into an 11-inch(ish) circle on a lightly floured surface. Transfer the dough to a baking sheet and spoon the filling into the middle of the circle, leaving a 1 to 2 inch border of dough for the crostata's crust. Gently fold the dough up over the fruit, pleating the edges to make them stronger.

★ **SMALL RECTANGLES:** Roll out the dough with a rolling pin or use your hands to flatten and pinch the dough into small rectangles. Have kids place the filling on the lower half of each rectangle, leaving about a ¼-inch border. Fold dough over each fruit filling and have kids press the edges well to seal. Cook on a baking sheet.

★ **SMALL CIRCLE:** Roll out the dough with a rolling pin or use your hands to flatten and pinch the dough into small circles. Using your clean hands, a cookie cutter, or the lid of a jar, punch muffin-sized circles out of the dough. Shape the dough circles into the wells of a muffin pan and add the fruit filling to the center

bake+bubble+cool

Bake the crostata for 20 to 25 minutes, until the crust is golden-brown and the fruit filling is tender and bubbling. Remove from the oven and let cool for 5 minutes. Sprinkle the tops with sugar before serving if you like! Serve warm or at room temperature. Say *Buon appetito*!...Enjoy your meal!

High Tea English "Crumpets"
+ Assorted and Savory Butters
+ Quickest Fruit Jam
+ Proper Tea

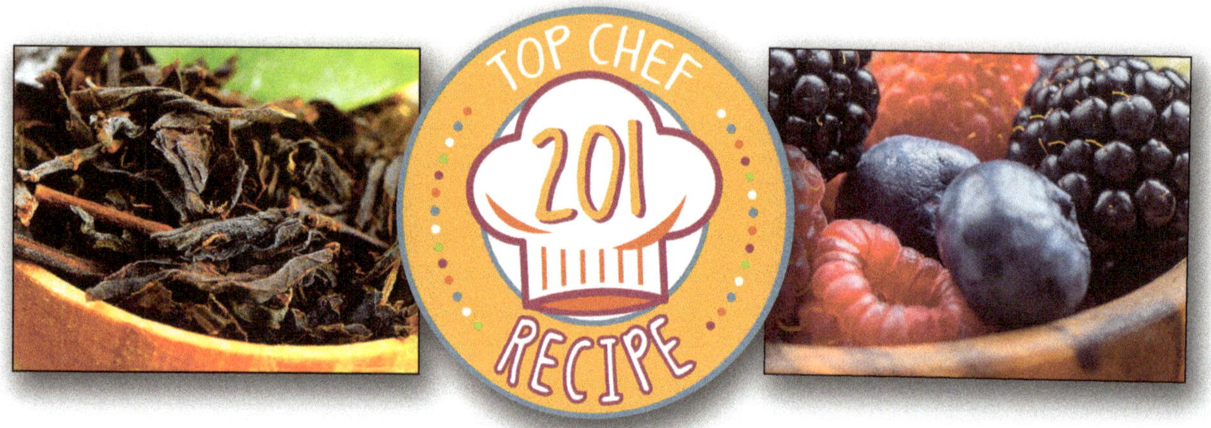

high tea english "crumpets"

ingredients

1 C whole milk
1 packet active dry yeast
1 T sugar
butter (for greasing pan)
1¼ C all-purpose flour
1 tsp salt
½ C sparkling water
½ tsp baking soda

mix+rest

Heat **1 cup of milk** until it is lukewarm. To a medium bowl, add the warm milk, **1 packet of yeast,** and **1 tablespoon of sugar** and let rest 10 to 20 minutes.

grease+preheat

Generously grease the wells of a muffin pan with **butter** and place the muffin pan in the oven while it preheats to 350 degrees F.

add+mix+rest

In a separate mixing bowl, add **1¼ cups of flour** and **1 teaspoon of salt**. Encourage kids to mix the dry and wet mixtures together until well combined. In a small bowl, stir a ½ cup

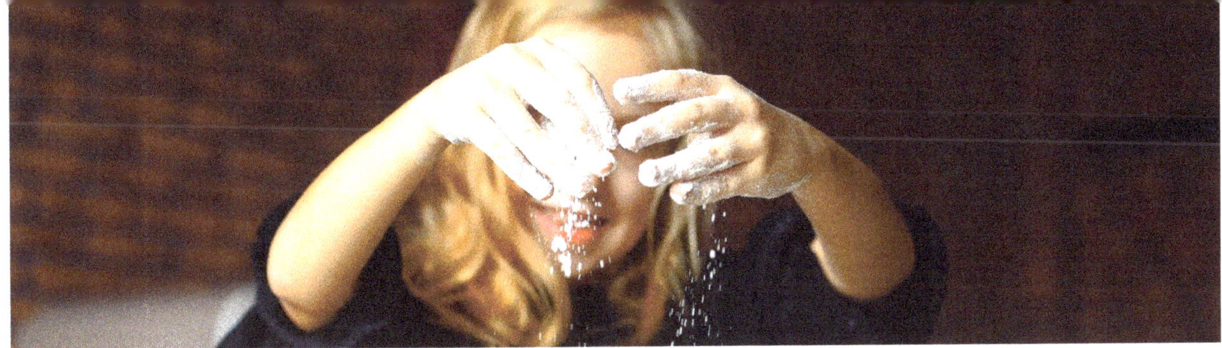

of sparkling water and ½ **teaspoon of baking soda** until dissolved and add to your bowl of batter, mixing to combine. Let rest at room temperature for at least 20 minutes or until the batter doubles in size.

pour+bake+toast

Remove the warmed muffin pan from the oven and then fill the wells ½ full with crumpet batter. Bake crumpets for 20 to 30 minutes, or until they are cooked through. Once your crumpets have baked, set your oven to "broil" and toast the tops golden brown. Careful—they will toast fast and can burn easily.

*To make crumpets gluten-free: Mix **1 packet of yeast** with **2 tablespoons of sugar**, **1 egg**, and **1 cup of milk**. Let rest and then add **1½ cups of gluten-free flour** and **1 teaspoon of salt**. In a separate bowl, mix together **1 cup of sparkling water** with ½ teaspoon of baking soda and add this mixture to the bowl of batter. Let rest for 20 minutes. Bake for 20 to 30 minutes until crumpets are cooked through, then toast them by turning the oven to "broil" until tops are golden brown. To make crumpets gluten and egg-Free: Substitute **1½ teaspoons of olive or grapeseed oil, 1 teaspoon of baking powder,** and **1½ tablespoons of water** for the egg.*

quickest fruit jam

ingredients

½ to 1 C fresh or frozen (thawed) berries
1 T sugar/maple syrup/honey
pinch salt

add+mash

There are two methods we suggest for mashing the berries into jam while they macerate: with a potato masher or with a resealable plastic bag!

For the potato-masher method, add ½ **to 1 cup of berries** to a mixing bowl, chopping larger berries first to make them easier to mash. Add **1 tablespoon of sugar/maple syrup/honey** and a **pinch of salt**. Using a potato masher, mash berries until you have a smooth consistency. Some small chunks are delicious! For the bag method, chop your berries and add to a resealable plastic bag with sugar and salt, seal tightly, and have kids squish with their hands until berries are mashed!

assorted sweet & savory butters

ingredients

sweet butters:
½ stick butter
1 tsp sugar/maple syrup/honey (+ more to taste)
suggested add-ins try 1 or more combos or make up your own:
brown sugar + cinnamon or pumpkin spice
orange zest + dried cranberries
cocoa powder + more sugar + peppermint extract or minced fresh mint
honey + vanilla extract
strawberries + orange zest

savory butters:
½ stick butter
¼ tsp salt (+ more to taste)
⅛ tsp pepper
suggested add-ins try 1 or more combos or make up your own:
fresh chives + parsley + lemon zest
Parmesan cheese + fresh basil + fresh sweet corn
lemon + capers
chopped tomato + basil

divide+zest+chop

Cut **1 stick of butter** in half. Choose your ingredients and separate them into "sweet" and "savory" categories. Zest any citrus fruit you've chosen and chop any veggies, fruit, or herbs.

measure+add+mix 'n mash

To your sweet butter, add **1 teaspoon of sugar/maple syrup/honey** and any other sweet additions you've chosen. To your savory butter, add ¼ **teaspoon of salt to taste,** ⅛ **teaspoon of pepper,** and any savory additions you've chosen. Mix'n mash the butters separately until ingredients are all combined.

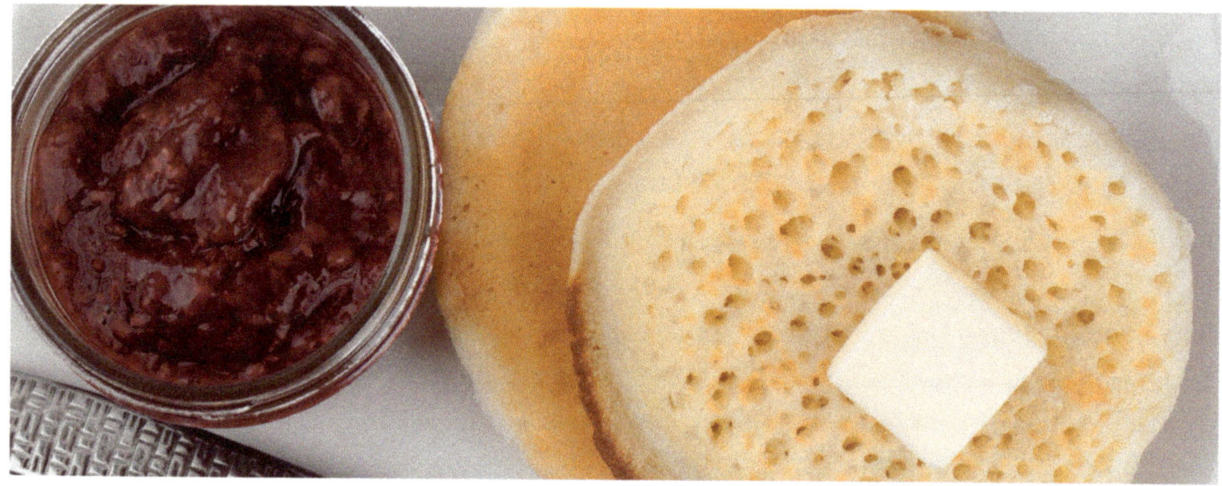

proper tea

ingredients

3 T sugar/maple syrup/honey
3 bags decaf black tea
½ C whole milk

boil+add+steep+pour!

Boil 3 cups of water in a saucepan. Add **3 tablespoons of sugar/maple syrup/honey** and stir until dissolved. Remove from heat and add **3 bags of black tea** and steep for 3 to 5 minutes. Add ½ **cup of milk**, pour, and enjoy!

Mealtime Chatter: How did your crumpets turn out? What other flavor jam do you want to make? Mango, peach? What wacky ingredients might you want to add to your butter?

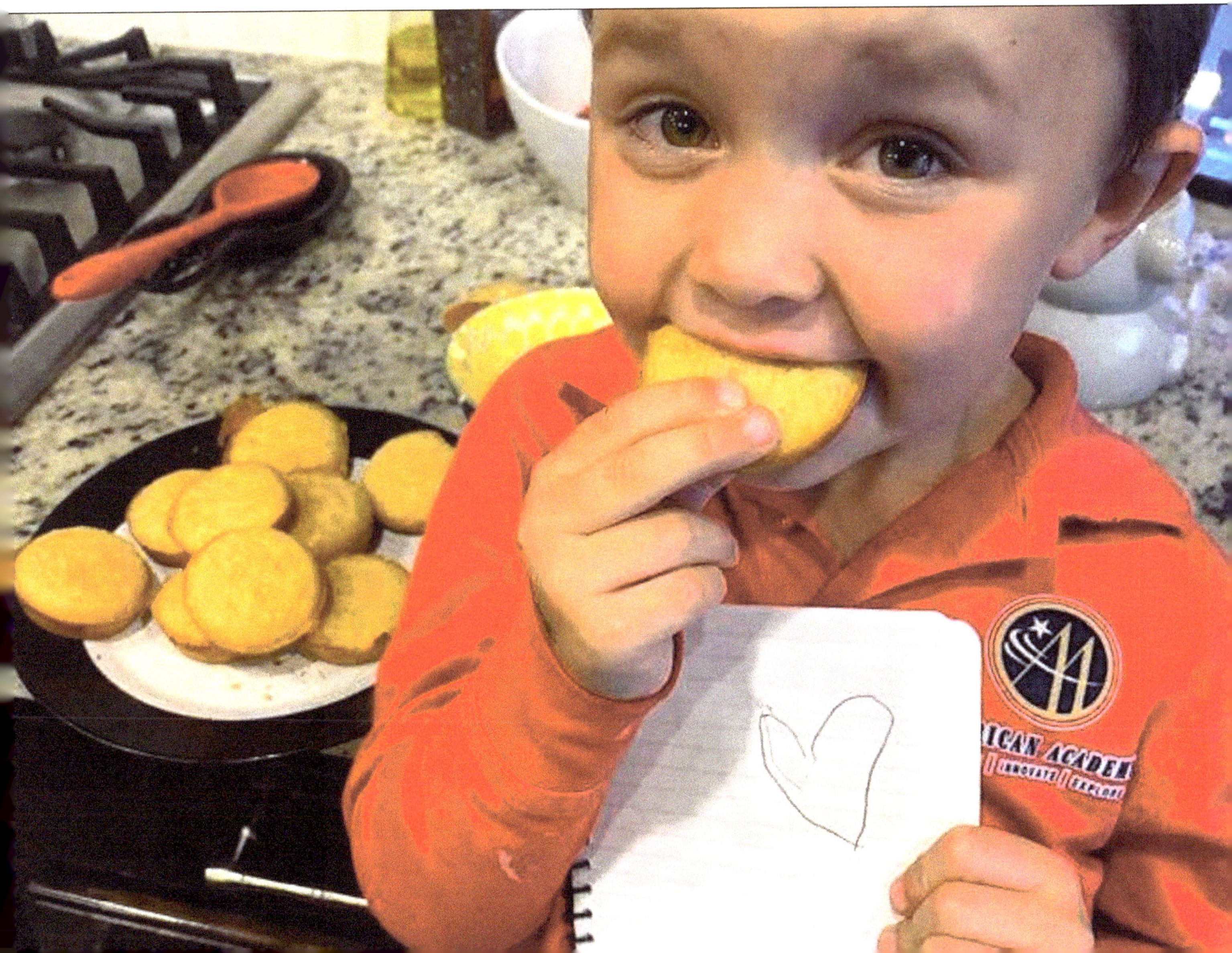

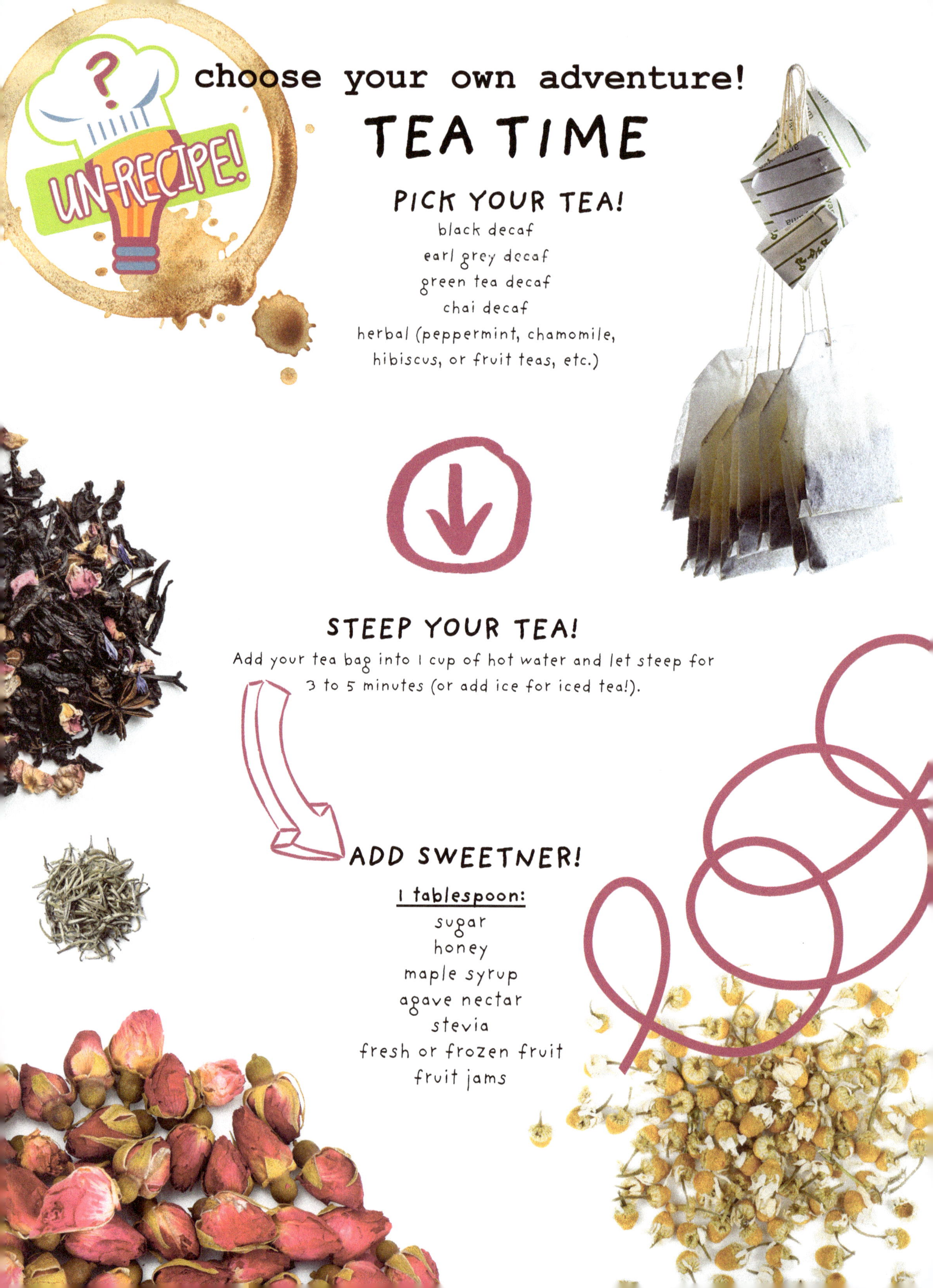

choose your own adventure!

TEA TIME

PICK YOUR TEA!

black decaf
earl grey decaf
green tea decaf
chai decaf
herbal (peppermint, chamomile, hibiscus, or fruit teas, etc.)

STEEP YOUR TEA!

Add your tea bag into 1 cup of hot water and let steep for 3 to 5 minutes (or add ice for iced tea!).

ADD SWEETNER!

<u>1 tablespoon:</u>
sugar
honey
maple syrup
agave nectar
stevia
fresh or frozen fruit
fruit jams

ADD EXTRA FLAVOR!

a pinch or splash:

cinnamon
pumpkin pie spice
cardamom
ground ginger
fresh mint leaves
vanilla extract
ginger juice

ADD CREAMINESS (if you want)!

(careful: some fruit teas will curdle with milk due to the acid content in some fruits)

1 tablespoon:

whole milk
coconut milk
cashew milk
soy milk
whipping cream
coffee creamer

CHEERS!

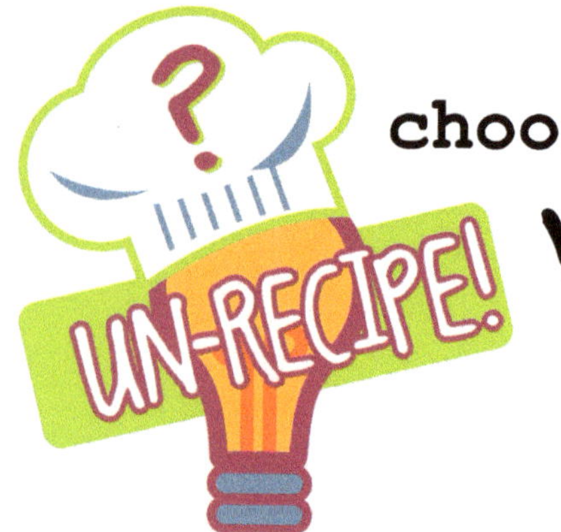

choose your own adventure!

WHIPPED CREAMS + COMPOTES

whipped cream base:

Pour **1 cup of heavy whipping cream** in a jar with a tight-fitting lid.

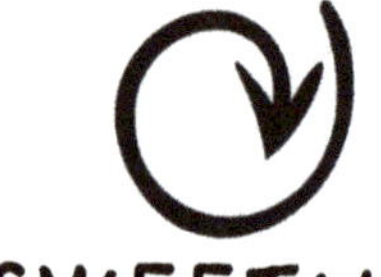

SWEETNER!

1 tablespoon:

powdered sugar
honey
agave nectar
maple syrup
a pinch of salt (surprisingly, salt makes things sweeter!)

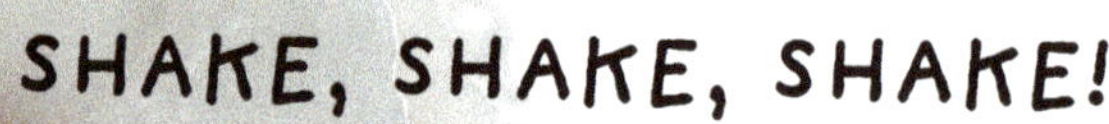

SHAKE, SHAKE, SHAKE!

Close the lid tightly and shake until a thick cream forms, about 3 minutes.

ADD FLAVOR!

to taste:

orange zest
lemon zest
lime zest
grapefruit zest
cinnamon
nutmeg
ginger
jam
cocoa powder
vanilla extract
brewed teas

MIX, DOLLOP, + ENJOY!

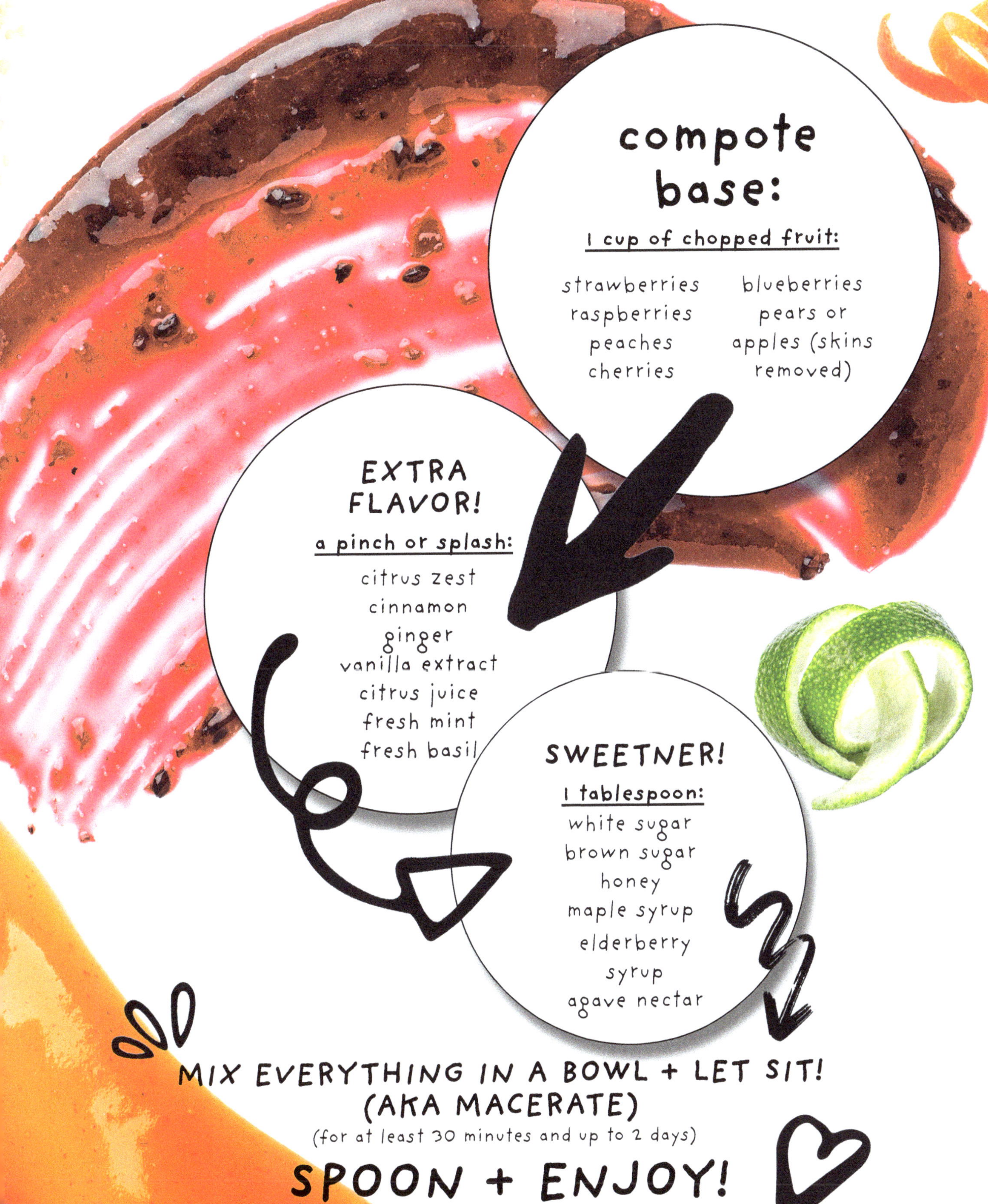

compote base:

1 cup of chopped fruit:

strawberries
raspberries
peaches
cherries
blueberries
pears or apples (skins removed)

EXTRA FLAVOR!

a pinch or splash:

citrus zest
cinnamon
ginger
vanilla extract
citrus juice
fresh mint
fresh basil

SWEETNER!

1 tablespoon:

white sugar
brown sugar
honey
maple syrup
elderberry syrup
agave nectar

MIX EVERYTHING IN A BOWL + LET SIT!
(AKA MACERATE)
(for at least 30 minutes and up to 2 days)

SPOON + ENJOY!

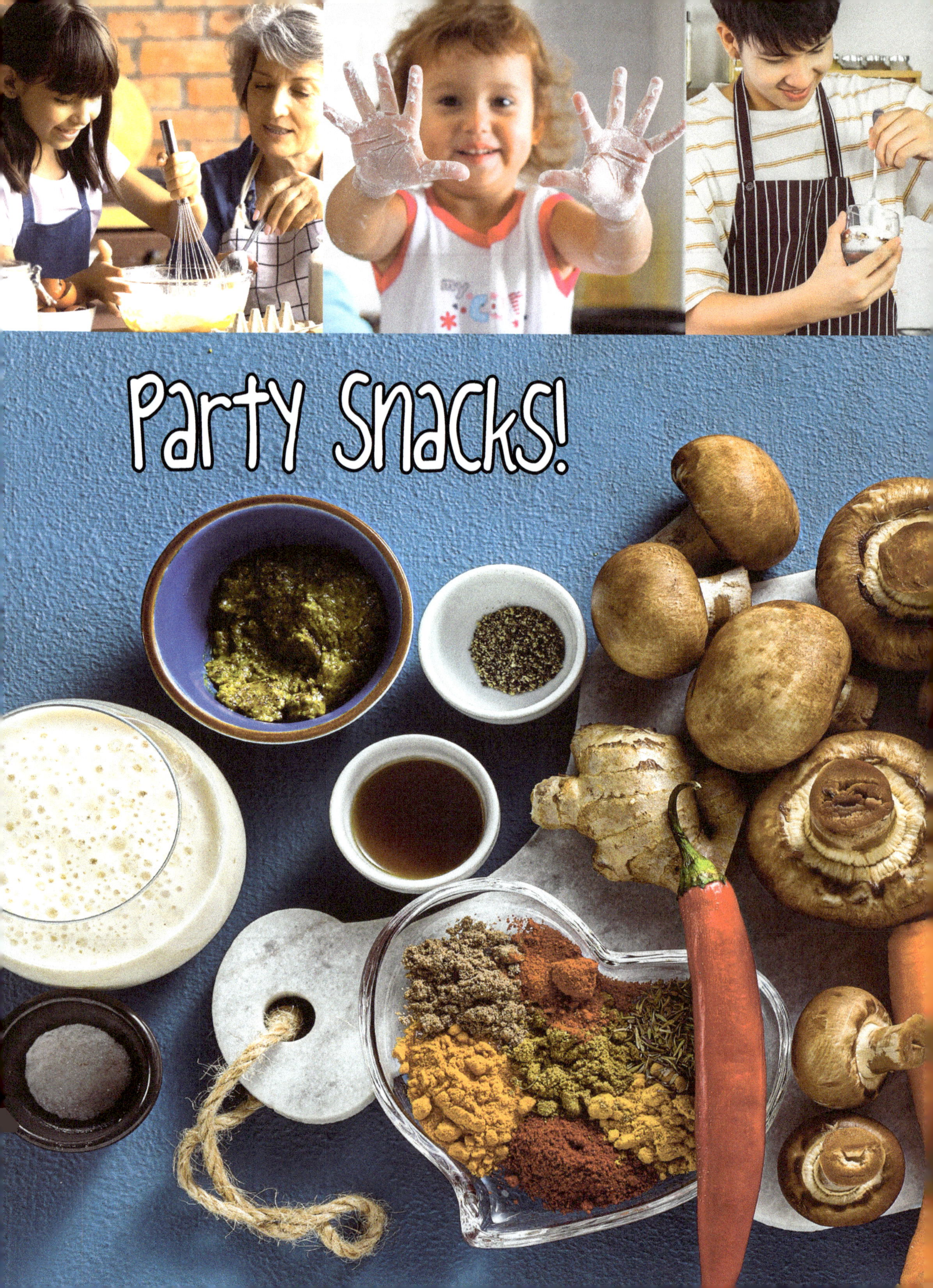

Party Snacks!

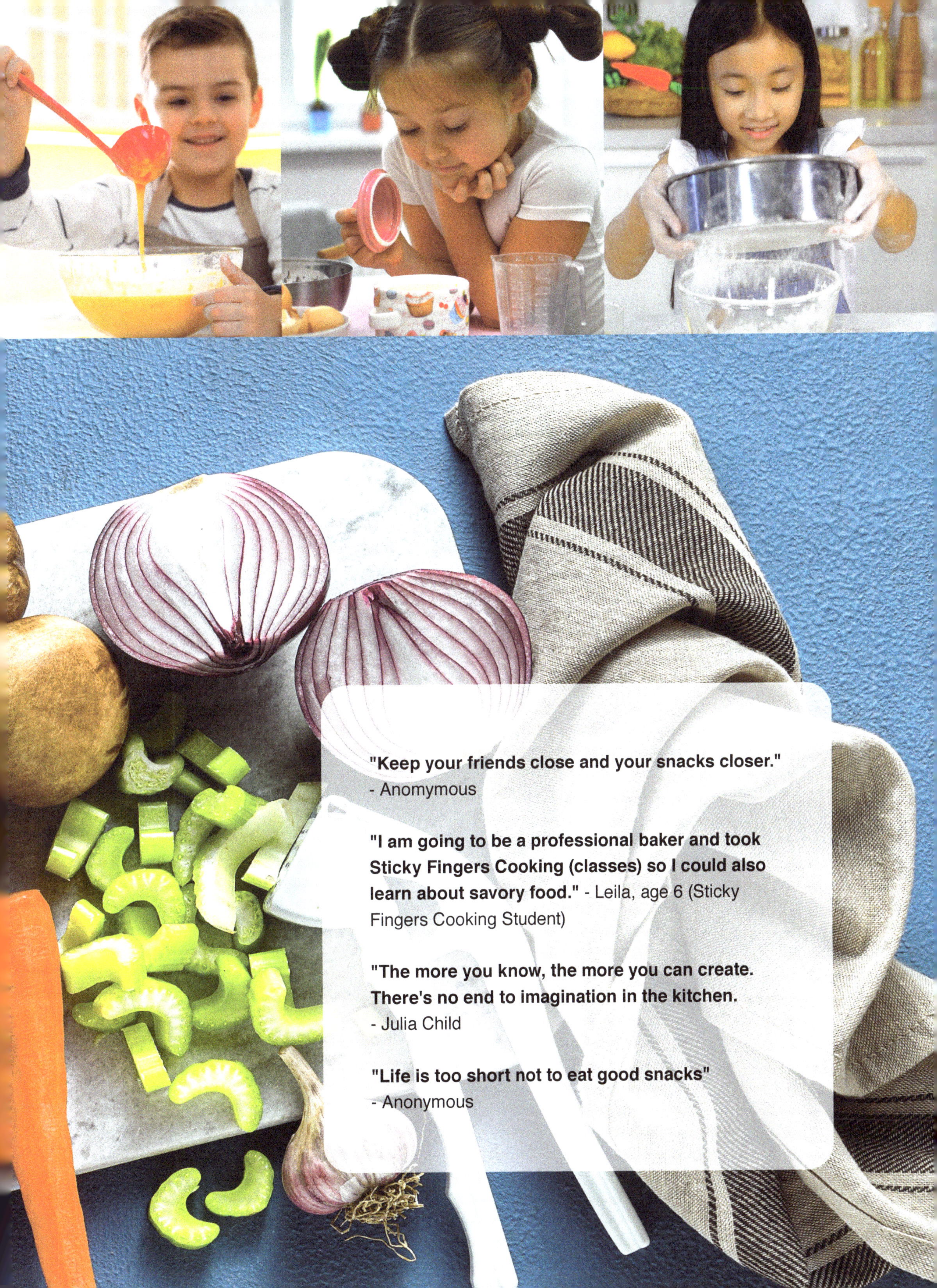

"Keep your friends close and your snacks closer."
- Anomymous

"I am going to be a professional baker and took Sticky Fingers Cooking (classes) so I could also learn about savory food." - Leila, age 6 (Sticky Fingers Cooking Student)

"The more you know, the more you can create. There's no end to imagination in the kitchen.
- Julia Child

"Life is too short not to eat good snacks"
- Anonymous

Golden Kale Pesto Crostini + Totally Tomato Bruschetta + Sweet Apple Ricotta Toast

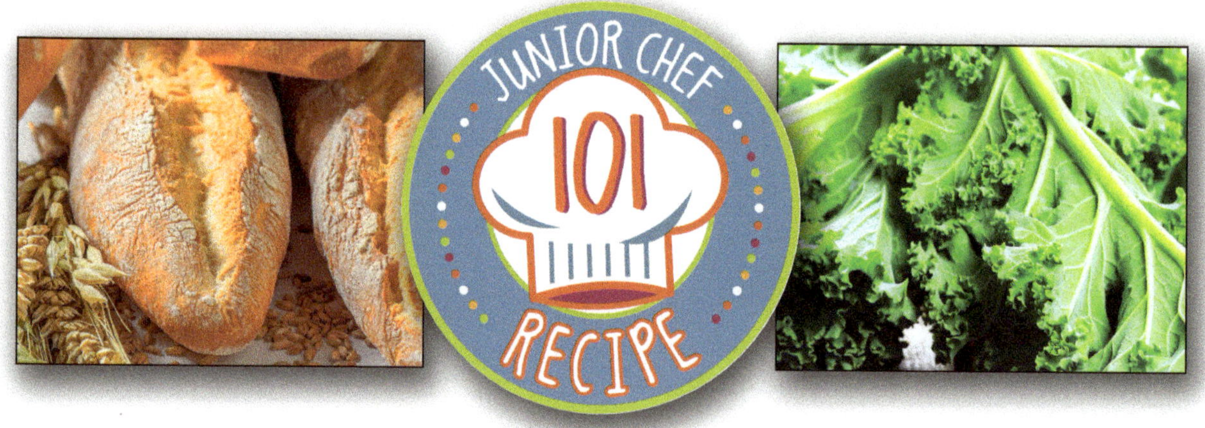

Bruschetta (brew-SKET-uh) is traditionally served in Italy as an antipasto, or starter course. There are many variations of bruschetta. Some simply have garlic rubbed on top of crisp bread and drizzled with olive oil while others include more elaborate toppings and flavorings. This recipe gives you sweet and savory options, so you can find your favorite way to eat this delicious dish!

golden kale pesto crostini

ingredients

1 fresh French baguette
olive oil (for drizzling)
pinche of salt

slice+drizzle+toast

Preheat your oven to 350 degrees F. On a slight angle, slice **1 baguette** into ¼ inch-thick pieces. Drizzle the crostini with **olive oil** and sprinkle with **pinches of salt**. Arrange crostini on a sheet pan and toast in the oven until lightly browned, about 3 to 5 minutes. Careful—they can brown quickly! Remove from oven and set aside to cool.

green kale pesto

ingredients

4 oz fresh green kale
1 garlic clove
½ lemon (juice)
¼ C sunflower seeds (sub green pepita seeds)
1 tsp sea salt
pinch pepper
¼ C olive oil
½ C pre-shredded Parmesan cheese (sub ⅛ C nutritional yeast)

chop+squeeze

Have kids remove the thick stems from **4 ounces of kale** and chop. Remove the skin of **1 garlic clove** and mince (cut into tiny, tiny pieces). Add kale and garlic into a blender or food processor. Using your hands or a citrus squeezer, squeeze the juice from ½ **a lemon** (for 1 teaspoon of lemon juice) and add into the blender.

measure+blend+slather

Continue adding the remaining pesto ingredients into your blender: ¼ **cup of sunflower seeds, 1 teaspoon of sea salt, a pinch of pepper,** and ¼ **cup of olive oil**. Cover your blender with the lid and blend everything together until thick and creamy, adding more oil or a little water to thin the pesto, if needed. Spoon the pesto into a small mixing bowl and add ½ **cup of Parmesan cheese**. Slather the beautiful *Green Kale Pesto* on your golden crostini toasts and serve with *Totally Tomato Bruschetta!*

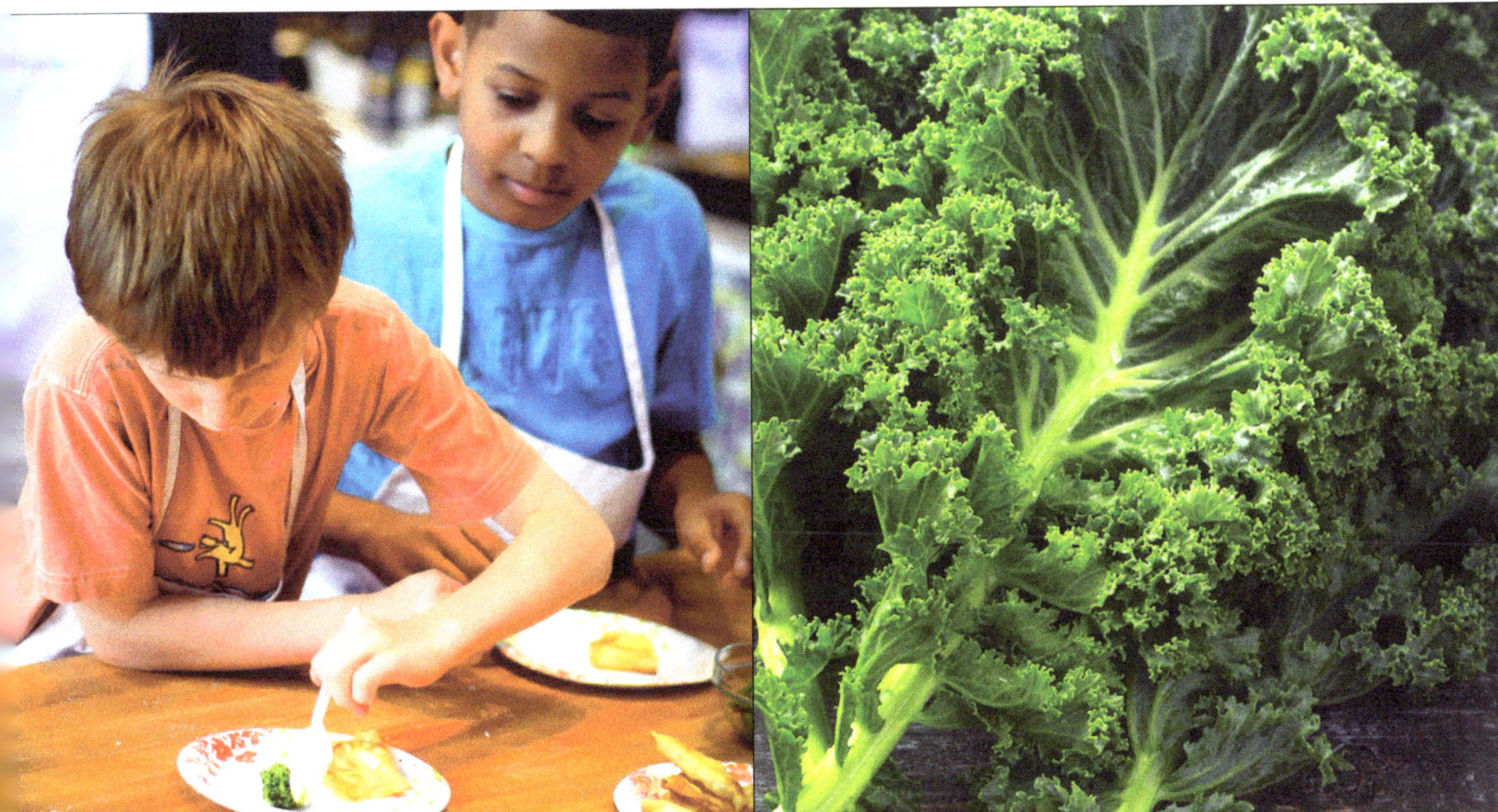

totally tomato bruschetta

ingredients

3 large tomatoes
½ lemon
pinch dried oregano
pinch dried basil
½ tsp sea salt
big drizzle olive oil

chop+squeeze+dollop

Slice 3 tomatoes in half and have kids chop them into tiny pieces. Add the chopped tomatoes to a small mixing bowl. Squeeze the juice from ½ lemon (for 1 teaspoon of juice) and add to the bowl along with a **pinch of dried oregano**, **a pinch of dried basil**, **½ teaspoon of salt**, and **a big drizzle of olive oil**. Stir well to combine and set aside to marinate. Dollop on top of the *Golden Kale Pesto Crostini!*

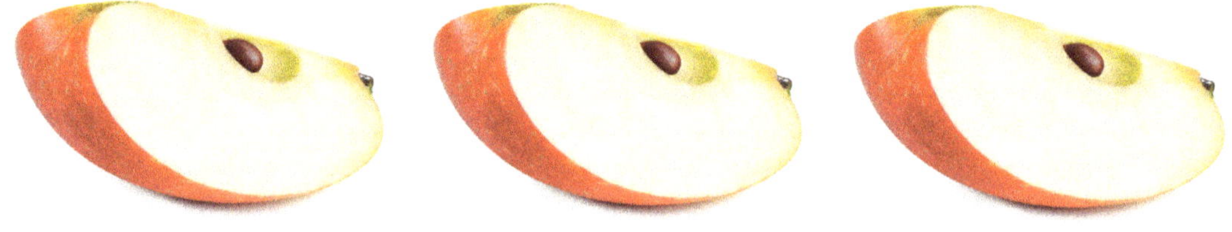

sweet apple ricotta toasts

ingredients

2 apples of your favorite variety
1 tsp lemon juice
pinch cinnamon
sugar or honey (to taste)
½ C ricotta cheese

chop+stir

Slice **2 apples** in half and have kids chop them tiny, tiny bits! Add the chopped apples to a small mixing bowl along with **1 teaspoon of lemon juice**, a **pinch of cinnamon**, and **a big sprinkling of sugar or drizzle of honey** to taste. Stir together and set aside for at least 10 minutes.

spread+drizzle+sprinkle+EAT!

Spread 2 teaspoons of **ricotta cheese** on each toast and top with the apple-cinnamon-honey mixture. Add another big sprinkling of sugar or drizzle of honey on top … ENJOY!

Kid-Made Cheesy Crackers

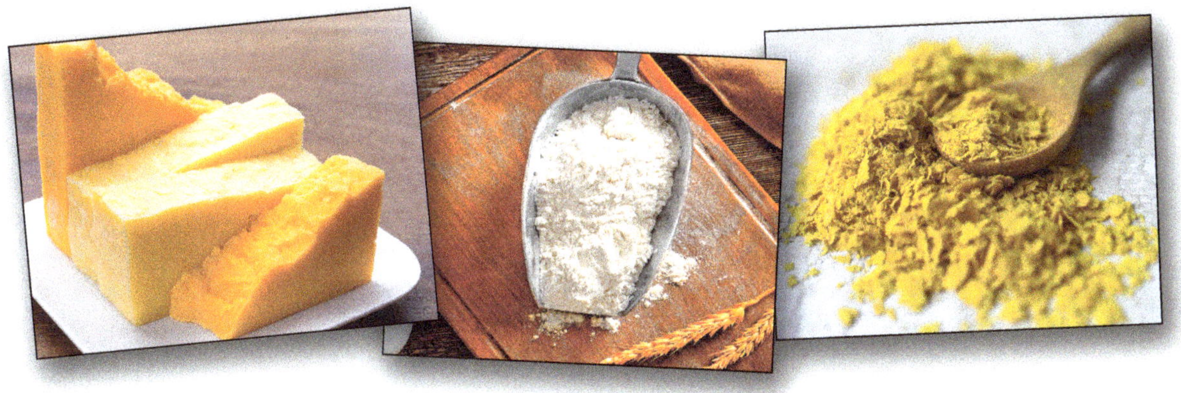

kid-made cheesy crackers

ingredients

6 oz cheese
¾ C all-purpose flour (+ more, if needed)
2 T cornmeal
½ tsp garlic powder
¼ C unsalted butter (softened)
1 T nutritional yeast

preheat+grate

Preheat your oven to 375 degrees F. Grate **6 ounces of cheese** and set to the side.

measure+combine

Measure ¾ **cup flour,** ½ **teaspoon salt, 2 tablespoons cornmeal,** and ½ **teaspoon garlic powder** in a large bowl and whisk to combine. Add grated cheese, soften ¼ **cup of softened butter**, and 1 tablespoon of cold water, and stir until a dough forms or blend in a food processor.

roll+cut

Sprinkle some flour on a cutting board or clean countertop and roll out the dough to an ⅛ of an inch. Using a knife or pizza cutter, cut dough into 1-inch squares. Use the flat end of a wooden skewer or a toothpick to poke a small hole in the center of each cracker.

transfer+bake

Carefully transfer your crackers to a lightly oiled or parchment-lined baking sheet and lay them out so they do not overlap. You can place them fairly close together. They will puff up but not spread much. Bake for 15 to 17 minutes or until puffed and edges start to brown. Sprinkle **1 tablespoon of nutritional yeast** over baked crackers. Let them cool completely and enjoy!

Baked Chiles Rellenos On-A-Stick

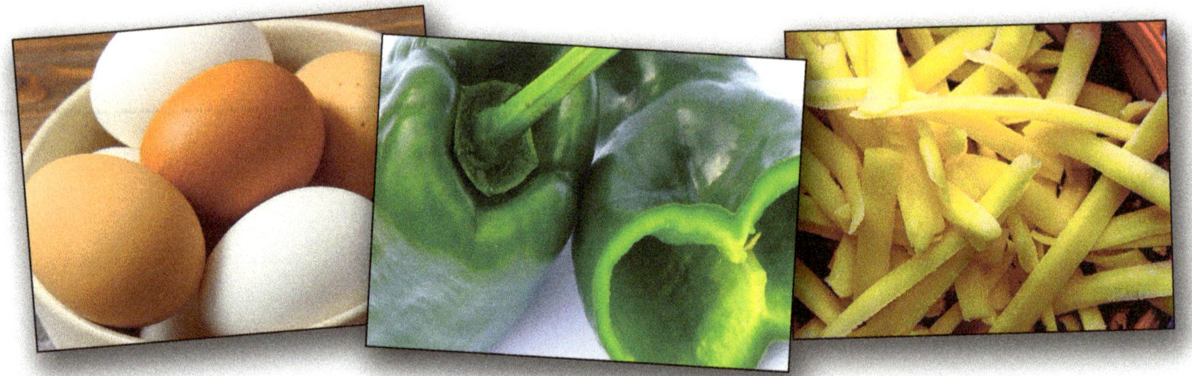

Chiles Rellenos (CHIH-lee-reh-YEH-no) is a traditional Mexican dish consisting of mild poblano peppers stuffed with meat or cheese and covered in an egg batter fried to golden perfection. It literally means "stuffed chile." Our version uses the same classic flavors but makes them bite-sized for easy snacking!

baked chiles rellenos on a stick

ingredients

your choice of pepper: 2 green bell peppers/8 oz can of whole mild green chiles/2 green poblano peppers
2 T + 2 T vegetable oil
pinch sugar
¼ tsp salt
2 eggs
8 oz jack cheese
¼ C all-purpose flour
½ tsp baking powder
¾ C milk
pretzel sticks or toothpicks (for serving)

preheat+chop

Preheat your oven to 375 degrees F. Remove the seeds and stems from **your choice of pepper** and chop them into tiny, tiny bits. Be careful to not touch your eyes or face while chopping (these chiles are very mild but can still irritate faces).

saute+brown

Warm a skillet on your stovetop to medium-high heat, add **2 tablespoons of oil** and the chopped chiles. Stirring frequently, cook until slightly browned, about 2 to 4 minutes. Then add **a pinch of sugar** and **¼ teaspoon of salt**.

crack+grate

While the chiles cook, crack and whisk **2 eggs** in a medium bowl. Grate **8 ounces of cheese** and add to eggs. Some prefer plain jack cheese for chiles rellenos and colby-Jack, cheddar, mozzarella, cotija, or Parmesan and yummy tool!

measure+whisk

Measure **¼ cup of flour, ½ teaspoon of baking powder, ¾ cup of milk,** and **2 tablespoons of oil** to the egg and cheese mixtures. And the cooked chiles and then whisk to combine.

bake+cool

Drizzle the wells of a muffin pan with the remaining oil and fill them halfway with the chile relleno mixture. Bake until the rellenos and puffed up, lightly golden brown and cooked through, about 20 to 30 minutes. Remove from oven and set aside to cool and firm up. Serve on **toothpicks** or **pretzel sticks** with creative toppings.

Here's some creative topping ideas!

- fresh torn cilantro
- fresh chopped tomatoes
- fresh lime juice
- sour cream
- corn
- chopped black olives
- mashed avocado
- mild salsa

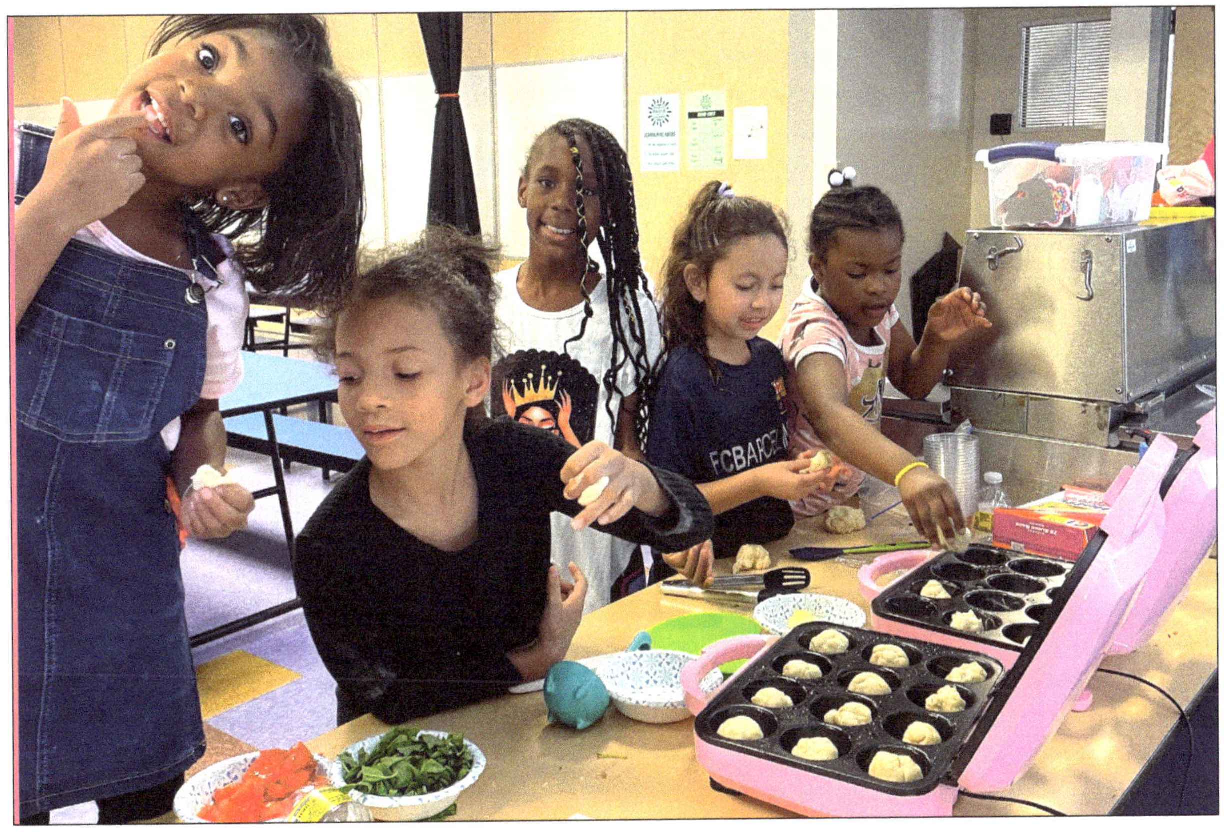

Quinoa Pizza Bites On-A-Stick + Italian Grape Ice

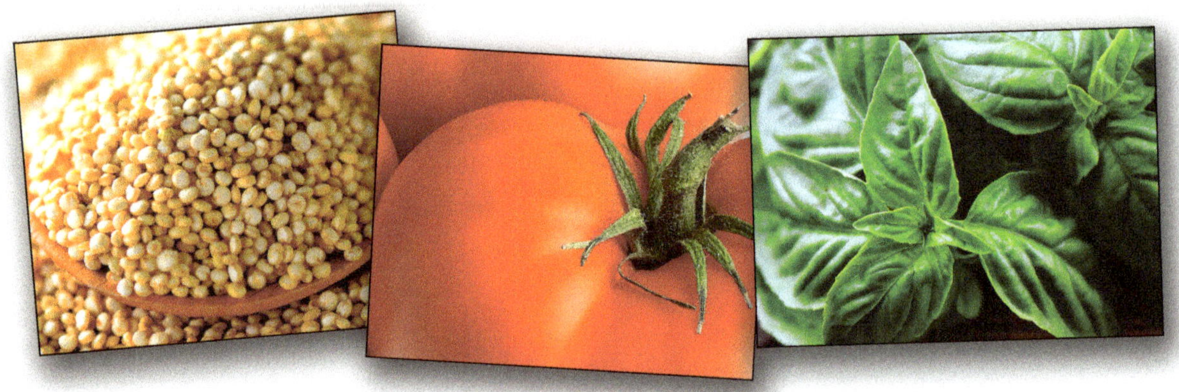

quinoa pizza bites on a stick

ingredients

1 C quinoa
3 large tomatoes
½ small white onion (sub 2 green onions)
1 small garlic clove
1 tsp olive oil
½ cup fresh basil (sub 2 tsp dried)
1 C smoked mozzarella cheese
½ tsp sea salt
1 tsp paprika
1 tsp oregano
2 large eggs
popsicle sticks
1 jar pizza sauce (for dipping)

rinse+boil+simmer+fluff

To prepare the quinoa, have kids vigorously rinse **1 cup of quinoa** (uncooked) in a fine mesh strainer (quinoa can be bitter! This will remove any bitterness on the outside hull). Place the quinoa in a saucepan with 1 cup of water on the stovetop and bring to a boil, then reduce to a simmer and cover with the lid. Cook 15 minutes, let sit 5 minutes, and then fluff with a fork. This will yield 2 cups of cooked quinoa for your pizza bites!

preheat+chop+squeeze

Preheat your oven to 400 degrees F. Have kids chop **3 tomatoes**. Over a large bowl, squeeze out all the juice and put the tomatoes aside for later use. Discard the tomato juice.

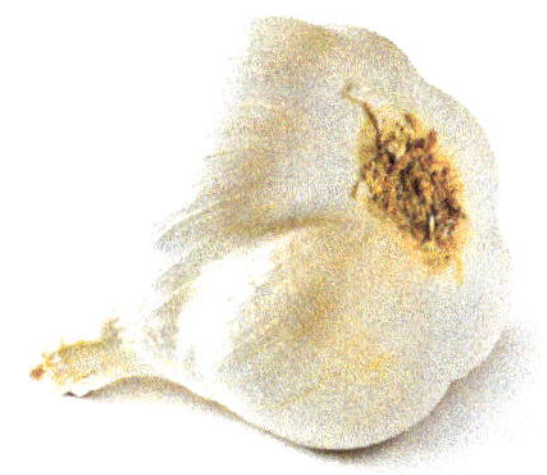 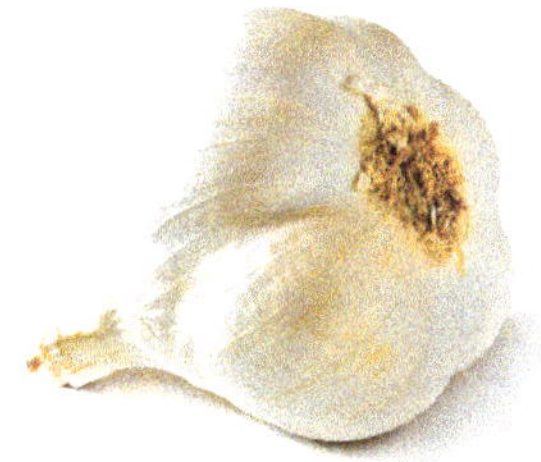 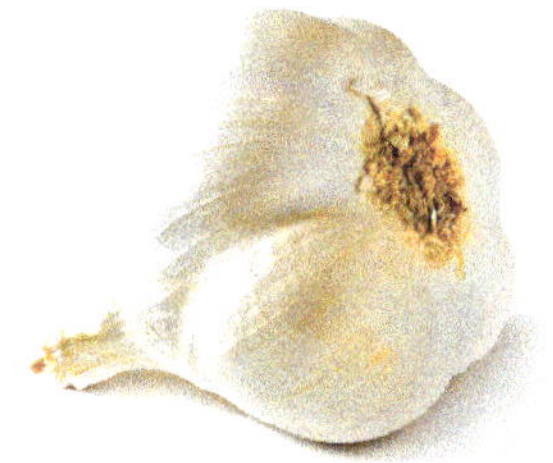 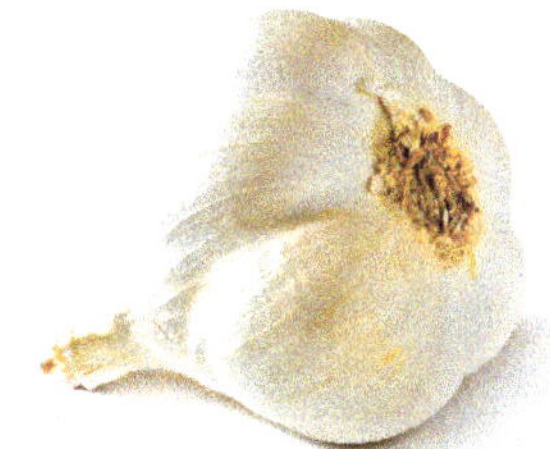

chop+sauté

Have kids chop ½ **of a white onion** into small pieces and mince (cut into tiny, tiny pieces) **1 garlic clove**. Heat a skillet on the stovetop to medium heat and sauté onions and garlic with 1 teaspoon of olive oil until soft and fragrant, about 1 to 2 minutes. Add your reserved tomatoes to the skillet and cook until warmed. Set aside.

grate+crack+measure+mush

If using **fresh basil**, remove the leaves from the stems and chop (or rip) into tiny pieces. Kids can grate **1 cup of mozzarella cheese** and add to a large mixing bowl along with a ½ **cup of basil,** ½ **teaspoon of sea salt, 1 teaspoon of paprika,** and **1 teaspoon of oregano**. Over a separate small bowl, crack **2 eggs**, remove any shells that may have fallen in, and then add the eggs to the mixing bowl with the cheese mixture. Stir to combine. To the same bowl add the cooked tomatoes, onions, garlic, and 2 cups of your cooked quinoa. Use a spatula to mush everything together!

scoop+roll+bake+EAT!

Scoop 2 tablespoons of the quinoa mixture and roll into a ball with clean hands. Repeat until all the quinoa mixture has been used. Arrange all the pizza balls ½ inch apart from each other on a sheet pan. Bake until bubbly and crisp on the outside and remove from oven. Let cool slightly. Have kids gently push a **popsicle stick** into each pizza bite and serve with your favorite jarred pizza sauce! *Mangiare la pizza* (man-JAR-ah lah PIZ-zah) … "Eat your pizza" in Italian!

italian grape ice

ingredients

½ to ¾ C sugar (or sub 4 packs of stevia)
1 C frozen white grape juice concentrate
1 T lemon juice

measure+blend

Into a blender, have kids pour 1 cup of water, a ½ **to** ¾ **cup of sugar, 1 cup of juice concentrate,** and **1 tablespoon of lemon juice**. Cover with the lid and blend until smooth! Serve in tall glasses with spoons or straws—ENJOY!

Carroty Soft Pretzel Bites
+ Crazy Carrot Cheese Dip

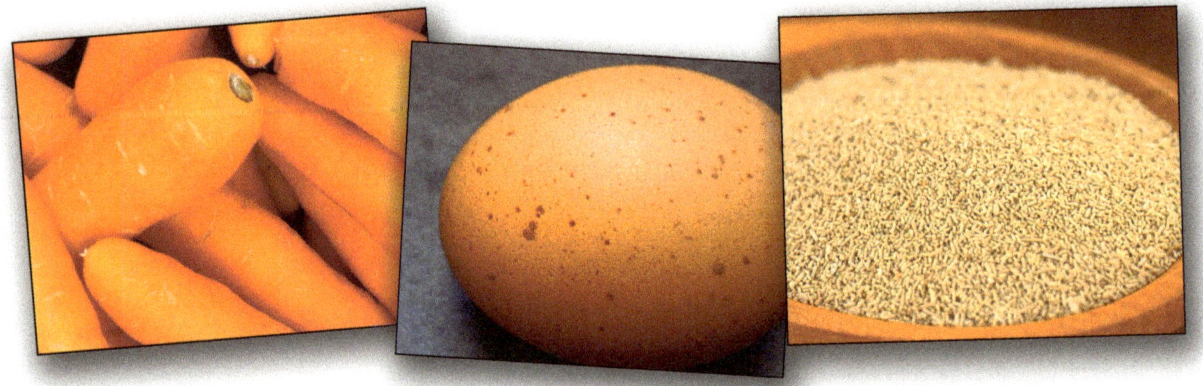

carroty soft pretzel bites

ingredients

1 package active dry yeast
1½ C lukewarm water
3 tsp honey/sugar
1 tsp salt
4 C all-purpose flour (more as needed)
2 carrots
1 egg
pinch of kosher salt (for sprinkling)

dissolve+combine

Dissolve **1 packet of yeast** and **1½ cups of lukewarm water** for 3 minutes. Then add in **3 teaspoons of sugar or honey**, **1 teaspoon of salt,** and **4 cups of flour**.

mix+rinse

Mix the dough together and set aside to rise for a 10 to 15 minutes. The longer it sits, the better the rise!

grate+separate

Grate **2 carrots**, one for the pretzel bites and one for the cheese dip. Separate the grated carrots into two equal piles.

preheat+knead

Preheat your oven to 435 degrees F and line a baking sheet with parchment paper. When the dough is ready, add half of the grated carrot and encourage kids to knead by hand for 5 to 10 minutes. Add flour as needed to reduce stickiness. Divide the dough into 12 sections and roll it out into long skinny snakes, ropes, or worms. As you work with the dough, it will become stickier. Keep adding flour as needed.

crack+brush+sprinkle

Crack **1 egg** and beat it in a small bowl. Once long dough snakes/worms have been rolled out, brush the dough with the beaten egg using a pastry brush. The egg makes the pretzels beautiful and shiny when they bake! Sprinkle top of the egg washed dough with just a little **kosher salt**.

shape+bake+dip

Shape your snakes/ropes/worms into a fun shape on the lined baking sheet. The shape doesn't matter; the pretzels will taste delicious no matter how they look! Slide the tray into the oven and bake for 8 to 10 minutes until golden brown.

ANY SWEET TREAT: Did you know a pinch of salt can actually make things taste sweeter?!

crazy carrot cheese dip

ingredients

1 tsp lemon juice (+ more to cook)
1 tsp kosher salt (+ more to cook)
3 big pinches pepper
2 T Greek yogurt or mayonnaise (or sub vegan mayonnaise)
¼ tsp honey/sugar (+ more to cook)
4 oz sharp cheddar cheese block
1 small carrot

measure+combine+grate

In a medium bowl, combine **1 teaspoon of lemon juice, 1 teaspoon of kosher salt, 3 big pinches of pepper, 2 tablespoons or yogurt or mayonnaise** and **¼ teaspoon of honey** or **sugar**. Grate **4 ounces of sharp cheddar cheese** and add to the same bowl. Set aside.

grate+cook+cool+mash

Grate **1 carrot**. In a medium nonstick skillet on your stovetop, combine grated carrots, a splash of lemon juice, a big pinch of salt, a drizzle of honey and 1 teaspoon of water. Cook the carrots over medium heat until soft, about 3 to 5 minutes, and let cool. Add the cooked and cooled carrots to the cheese bowl and encourage kids to toss and mash (with a wooden spoon or potato masher) until the cheese and carrots turn into a dip! Serve with your *Carroty Soft Pretzel Bites, YUM! YUM!*

Crispy Cheesy Corn Dog Bites on a Stick + Honey Mustard Dip + Summer Garden Pickles + Fresh Frozen Lemonade

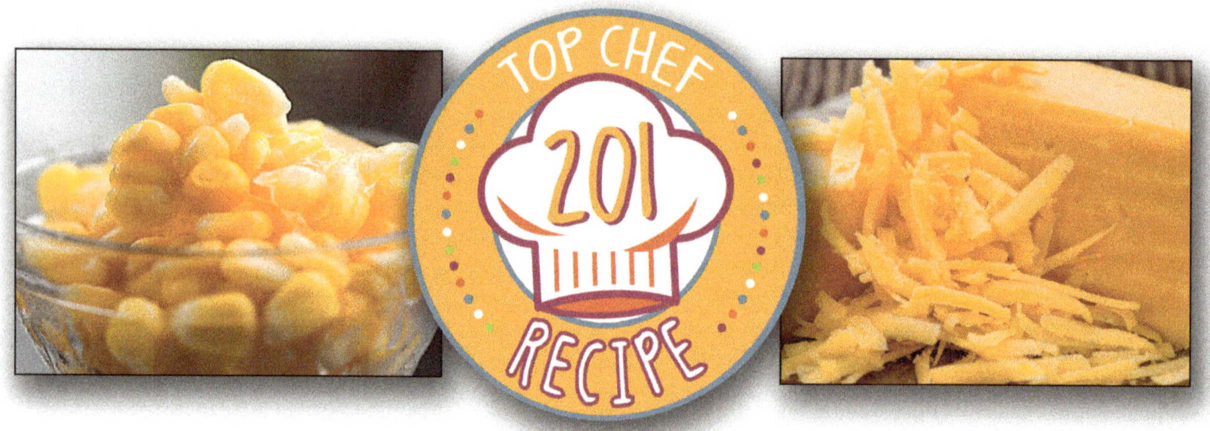

crispy cheesy corn dog bites

ingredients

olive oil
1 C yellow cornmeal
1 C all-purpose flour
1 tsp kosher salt
baking powder
1 tsp baking soda
1 C fresh, frozen (thawed) or canned (drained) corn
1½ C buttermilk
⅓ C grated cheddar cheese
6 veggie dogs
4 T cornstarch (for dredging)

preheat+measure+combine

Preheat your oven to 350 degrees F. Generously oil a muffin pan with **olive oil**. In a medium mixing bowl, measure and combine **1 cup of cornmeal, 1 cup of flour, 1 teaspoon of salt, 1 teaspoon of baking powder,** and ¼ **teaspoon of baking soda**.

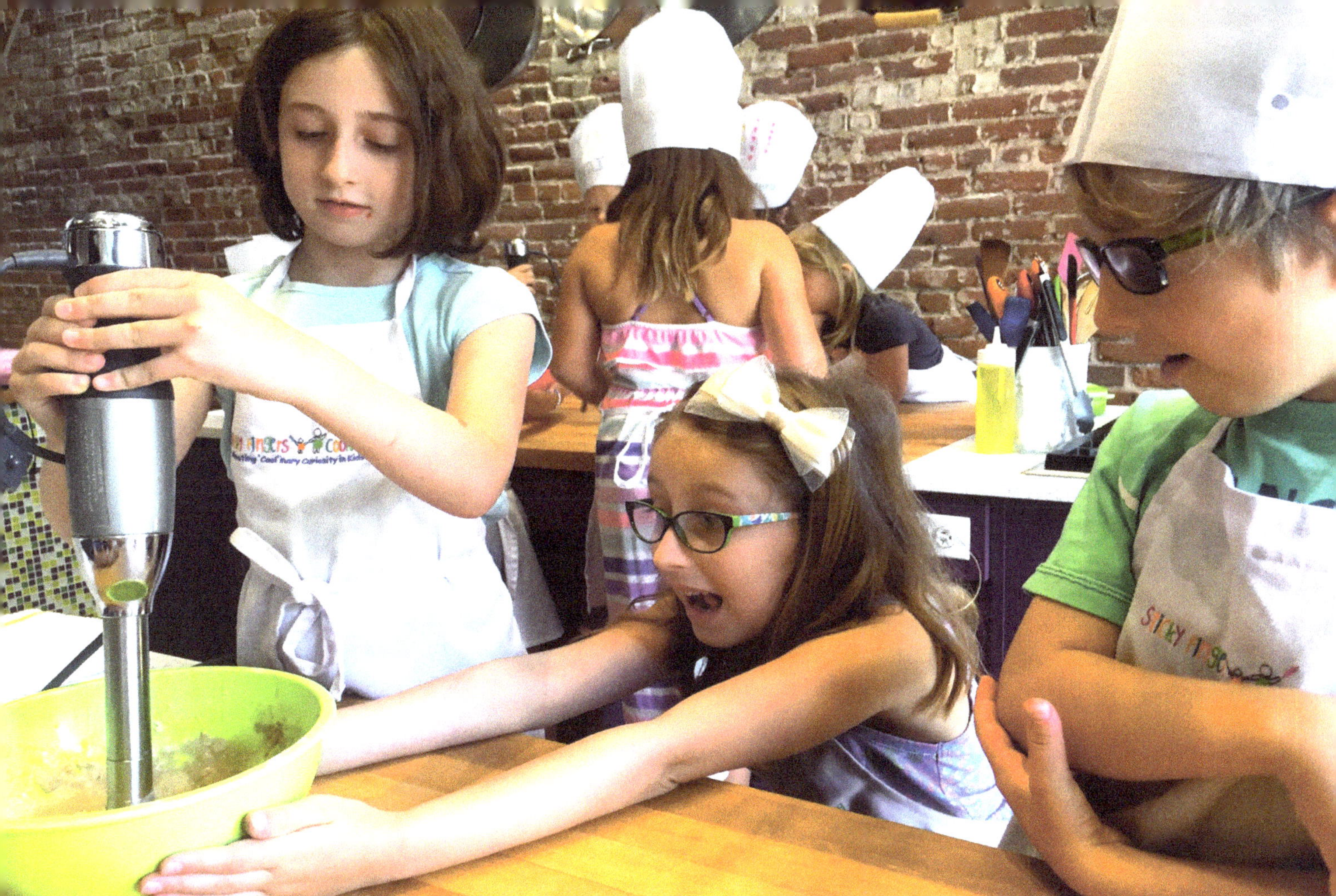

purée+greate

Using either a blender, food processor, or immersion blender and bowl, and combine **1 cup of corn** and **1½ cups of buttermilk**. Purée until smooth and then add **⅓ cup of cheese**.

add+stir+rest

Add the dry ingredients to the wet ingredients and stir tenderly, only enough times to bring the batter together (there should be some lumps!). Set aside to rest.

cut+roll+tap

Cut **6 veggie dogs** into bite-sized pieces, about 4 to 6 pieces per dog. Scatter **4 tablespoons of cornstarch** into a shallow bowl and roll each hot dog piece in cornstarch. Tap well to remove any excess cornstarch.

dip+cook+serve

Take each veggie dog bite and quickly dip it in and out of the batter and then immediately into your greased muffin pan wells. Bake about 10 to 15 minutes until the coating is golden brown and the tops are crispy. Remove corn dog bites from the oven and stick one toothpick into each bite to serve!

honey mustard dip

ingredients

3 T honey

3 T deli mustard

measure+whisk

Measure **3 tablespoons of honey** and **3 tablespoons of mustard** into a small bowl. Whisk until well combined.

summer garden pickles

ingredients

2 cucumbers
2 small carrots
¼ C fresh, frozen (thawed) or canned (drained) corn

¼ C white wine vinegar
½ C sugar
1 T salt
1 heaping tsp of pickling spice

slice+measure+whisk

Slice up **2 cucumbers** and **2 carrots** and add to a bowl with ¼ **cup of corn**. In a separate bowl, **measure** ¼ **cup of vinegar,** ½ **cup of sugar, 1 tablespoon of salt,** and **1 heaping teaspoon of pickling spice**. Whisk to combine.

pour+coat

Pour the pickling solution over the veggies and stir to coat. Set aside to pickle for at least 30 minutes and then enjoy!

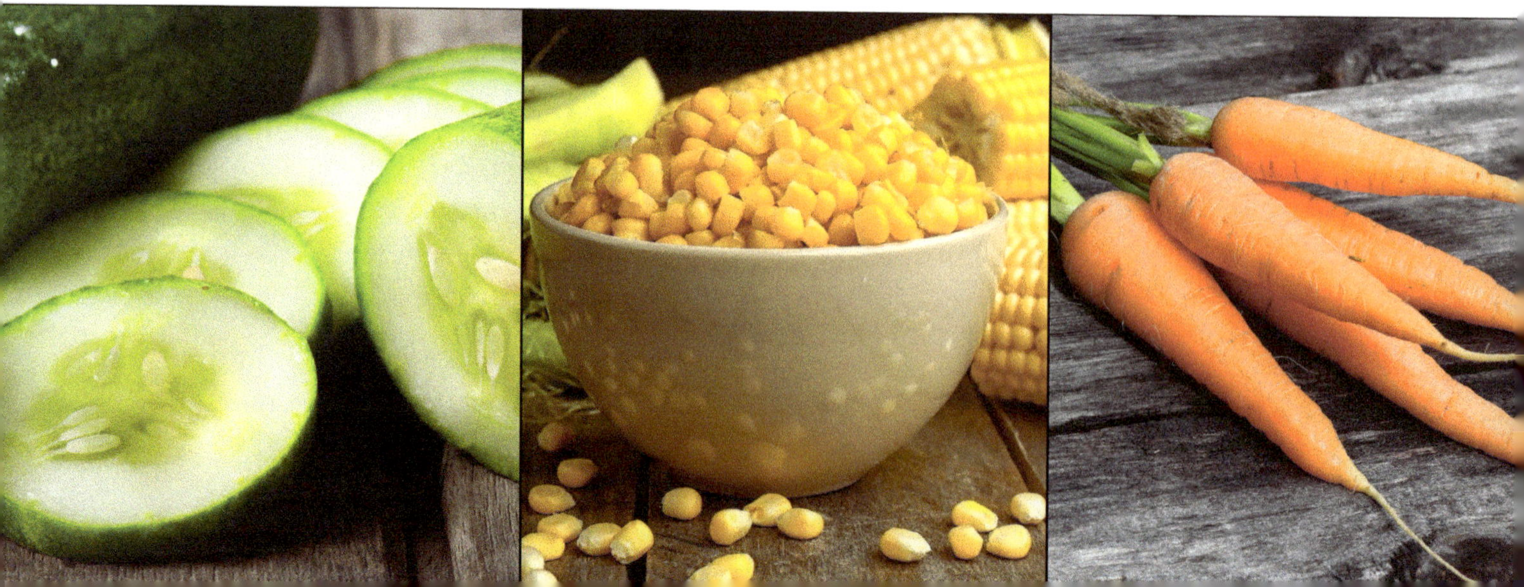

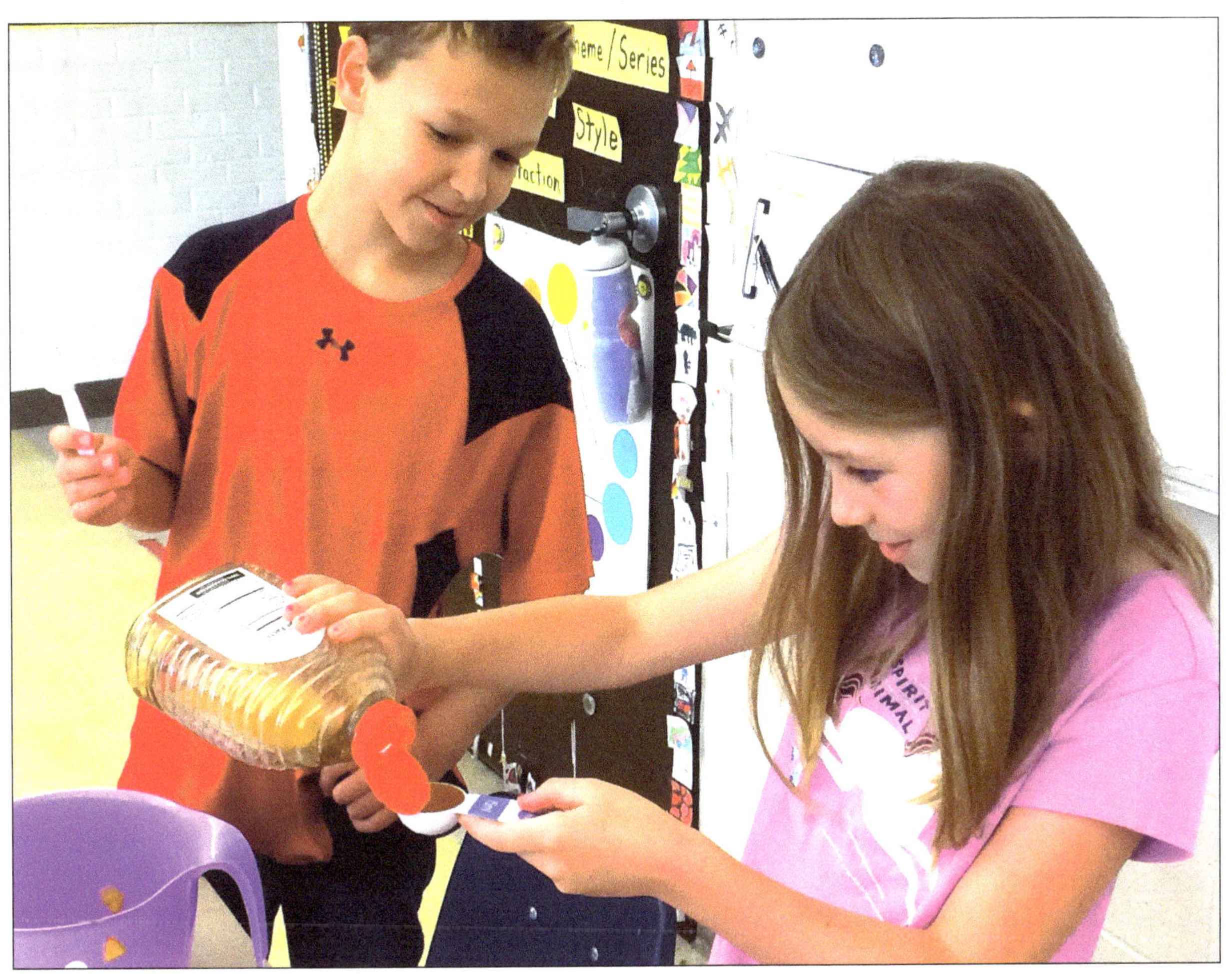

fresh frozen lemonade

ingredients

2 lemons
½ C sugar/honey (sub 2 to 3 packs of Stevia)
2 C ice

squeeze+add

Squeeze the juice of **2 lemons** into your blender or a pitcher for use with an immersion blender. Measure and add ½ **cup of sugar or honey**, 2 cups of water, and **2 cups of ice** to the blender pitcher.

purée+adjust+pour

Puree your lemonade until smooth. Does it need more lemon juice?? More sweetner? Adjust, serve, enjoy!

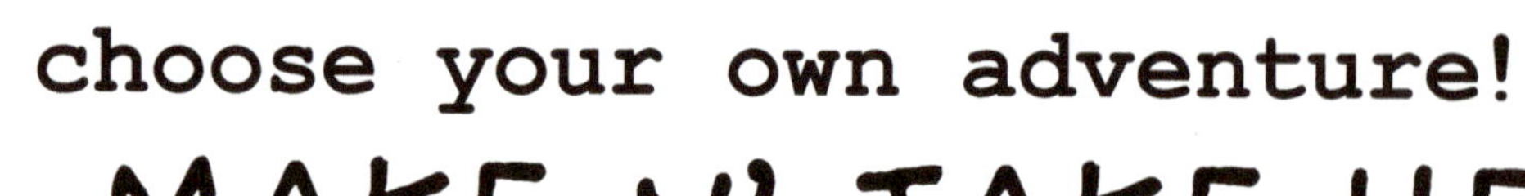

UN-RECIPE!

MAKE N' TAKE HEALTHY FAMILY PARTY MIX

party mix base!

Start by mixing **4 cups of oats** and **½ teaspoon of salt** in a large bowl. In a large skillet over low heat, melt a **¼ cup of butter with ½ a cup honey** or **maple syrup**. Once the butter and honey are melted, raise the heat to medium for 30 seconds to a minute, until the mixture gets bubbly. Reduce the heat to low, add the oats and salt, and stir for 3 to 5 minutes, or until the oats are nutty and fragrant. Set aside to cool.

pick sweet or savory add-ins!

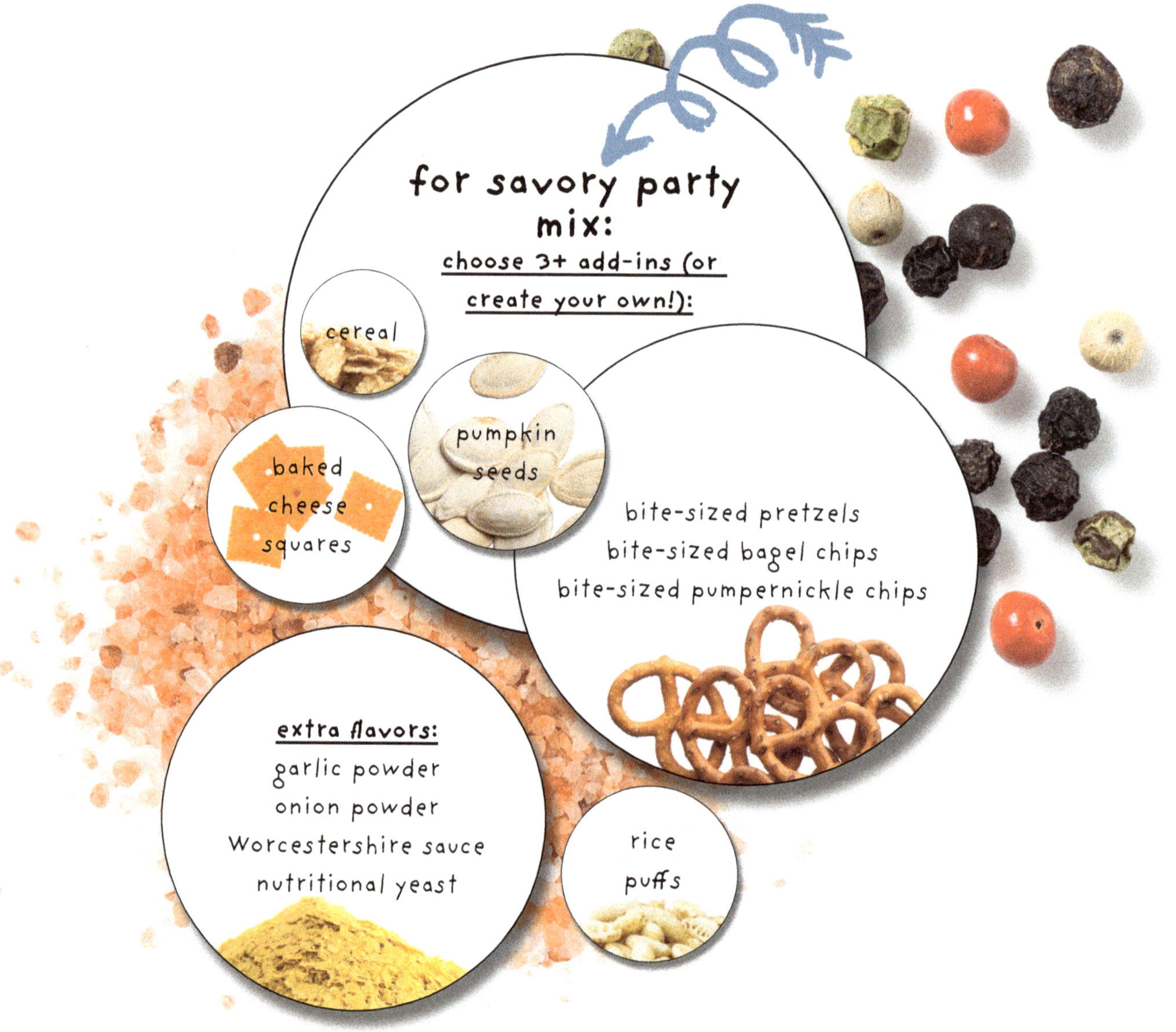

for savory party mix:

choose 3+ add-ins (or create your own!):

cereal

pumpkin seeds

baked cheese squares

bite-sized pretzels
bite-sized bagel chips
bite-sized pumpernickle chips

rice puffs

extra flavors:

garlic powder
onion powder
Worcestershire sauce
nutritional yeast

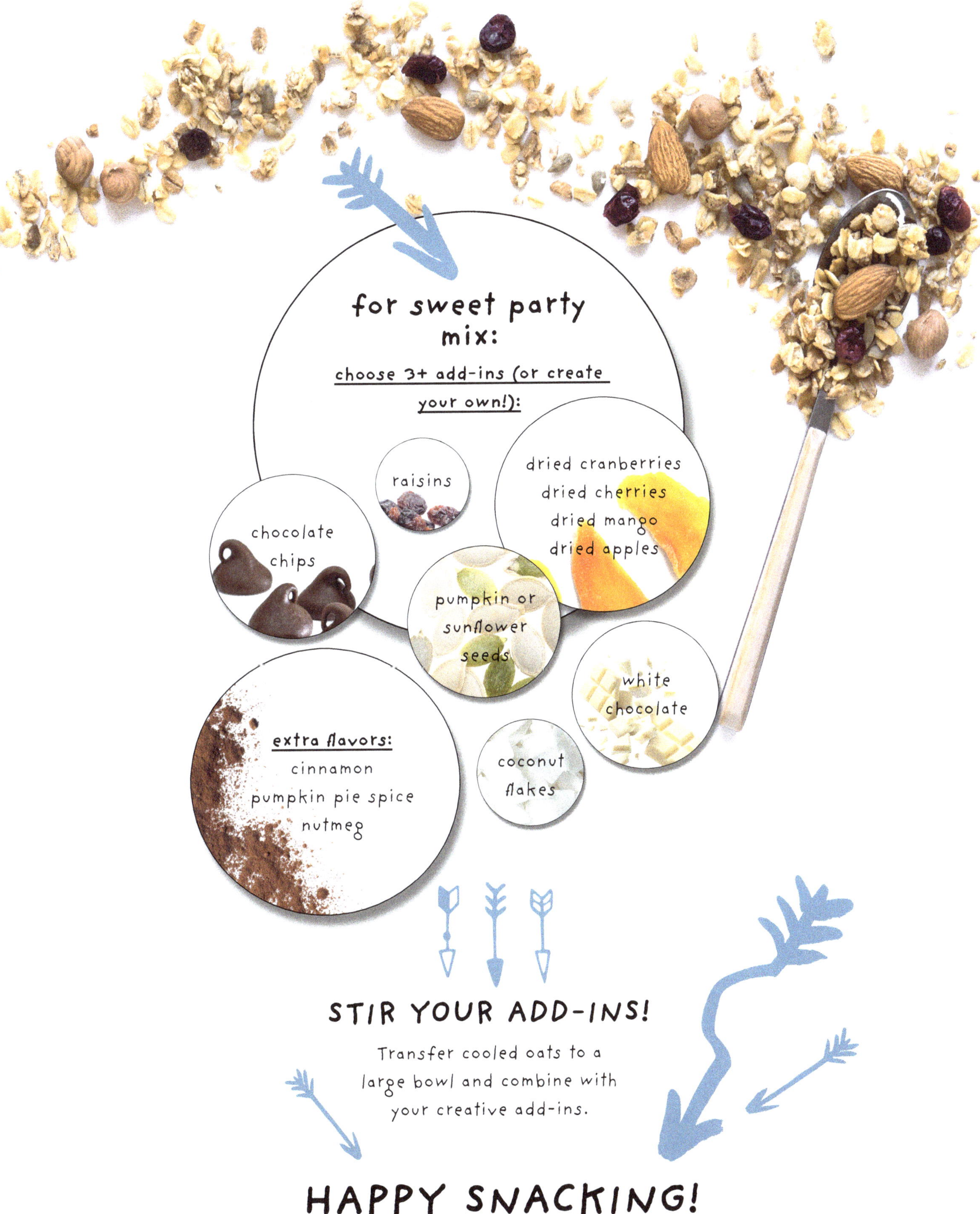
for sweet party mix:
choose 3+ add-ins (or create your own!):
raisins
dried cranberries
dried cherries
dried mango
dried apples
chocolate chips
pumpkin or sunflower seeds
white chocolate
extra flavors:
cinnamon
pumpkin pie spice
nutmeg
coconut flakes
STIR YOUR ADD-INS!
Transfer cooled oats to a large bowl and combine with your creative add-ins.
HAPPY SNACKING!

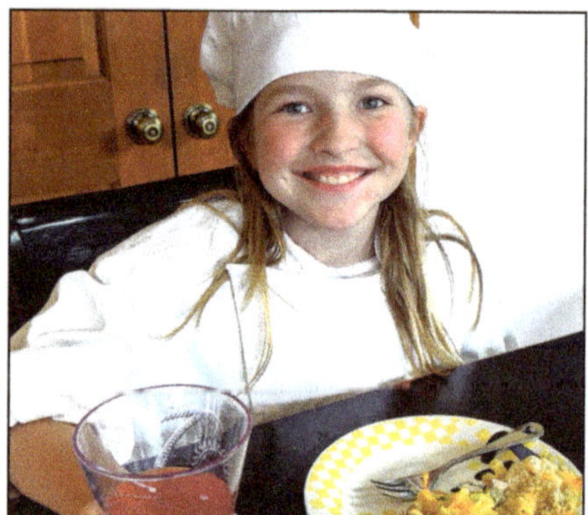

Congratulations to Young Chef Lily!

The Basic Training Baking Boot Camp Cover Star

How did you first get introduced to baking?
Response: My dad bakes a lot and honestly I just saw it as magic or something.

What have you learned from baking? What do you think it can teach kids?
Response: I've learned that baking is pretty much just science. I think it could teach kids proper kitchen use and some character.

Baking is considered to be very nostalgic because people are often reminded of their childhood. What memories do you have of baking or what moments do you think you'll treasure when you're an adult?
Response: Well, honestly, I'll have some memories from Sticky Fingers, of course! And the time I made the seven-layer cake. But sometimes it's hard to have memories of things you bake.

What advice do you have for junior chefs when it comes to baking in the kitchen?
Response: Always follow the directions because when it comes to baking, a little too much of something can go a long way! Whereas in cooking, you can modify the recipe a little, with baking you never want to do that.

What is your favorite ingredient to bake with?
Response: Probably the flavoring that goes in whatever you are baking.

Baking doesn't have to be just sweet; it can be savory as well! What's one of your very favorite savory dishes you like to bake?
Response: Sometimes I like to make lunch crepes with a long sausage inside and a tortilla on the outside.

If you could only eat one baked good for the rest of your life, what would it be?
Response: Banana bread because it has protein as well as a little banana for healthiness.

If you could have any baking superpower, what would it be and why?
Response: I would have to choose as soon as I mix the ingredients for what I'm going to bake, it immediately turns it to what I'm going to bake! The reason? So I could give some to family friends and strangers.

What's a favorite baking pun or joke of yours? No joke can be too cheesy for us ;)
Response: Wanna hear a pizza joke?...Nah it's too cheesy :)

P. S. you can call me Lily. It is my preferred nickname.

VERY GRATEFUL ACKNOWLEGMENTS

"I don't like tomatoes and I STILL love this!" *-Owen, age 10*
"Kale is my favorite!" *-Max, age 8* **"I would eat 100 of these!"** *-Amile, age 6*

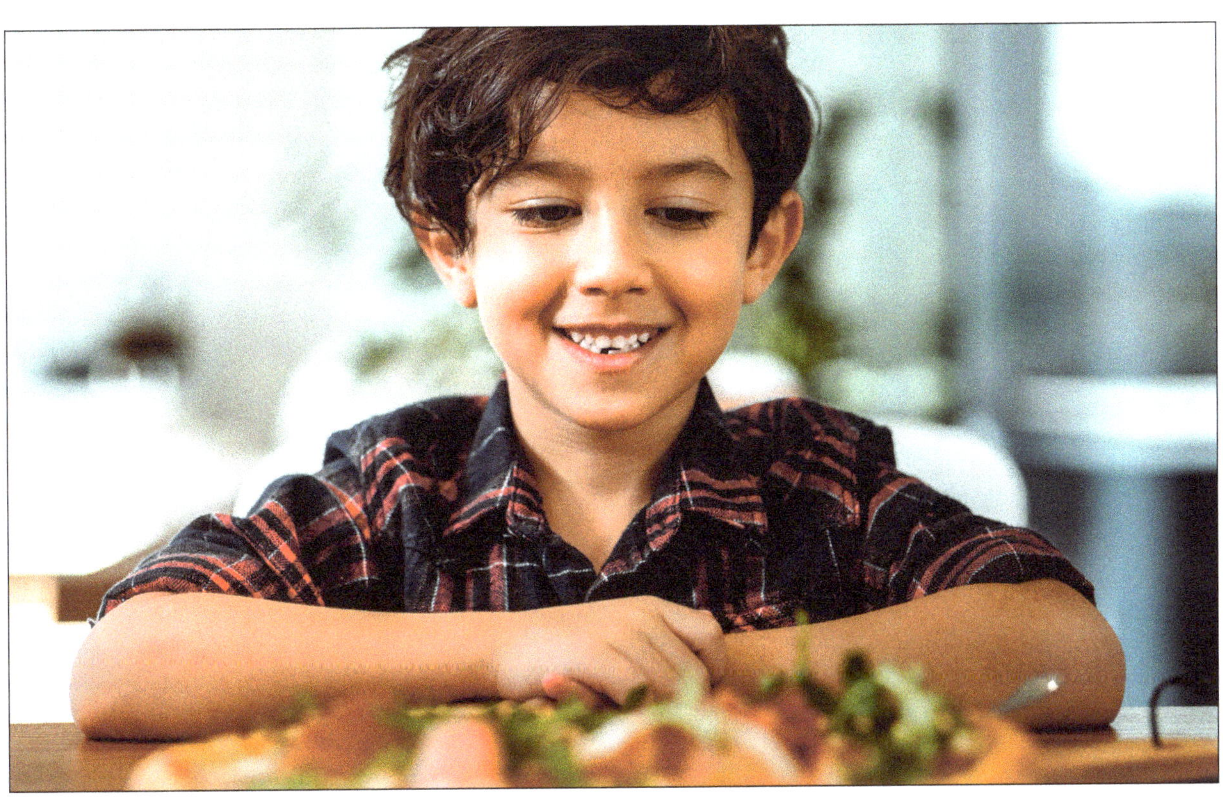

As always, thank you to each of our always amazing *Sticky Fingers Cooking* students. Your enthusiasm, optimism, and honest feedback that only a child can give keep us going strong. Keep cooking and keep taking WHISKS!

My family means the world to me. I am proud that my close and extended family and I, love and support each other every day. I am so lucky.

A massive thank you to our exceptional team of Chef Instructors who are the heart and soul of Sticky Fingers Cooking. Gratitude is given to Lilyana, and her family, for submitting her lovely photo for our cover. My most sincere and grateful acknowledgements to Emily Moore from Red Pen LLC, Amy & Peregrin Marshall of Web501, Jacqui Gabel, Jennifer Gauerke of YellowDog Denver, Shannon McLaughin, and the numerous photographers who each contributed to this delicious book for all awesome 'cool'inary kids!.

I'm profoundly thankful and in awe of our Sticky Fingers Cooking administrative team. Thank you to our creatively talented cookbook team; Joe Hall, Natasha McCone, Kate Bezak, and Francine Huang. Your united combination of enthusiasm, compassion, creativity, grit, wit, and steadfast attention to wondrously measure, knead, and bake the dough of success every year!

THE HANDY INDEX

About the Author

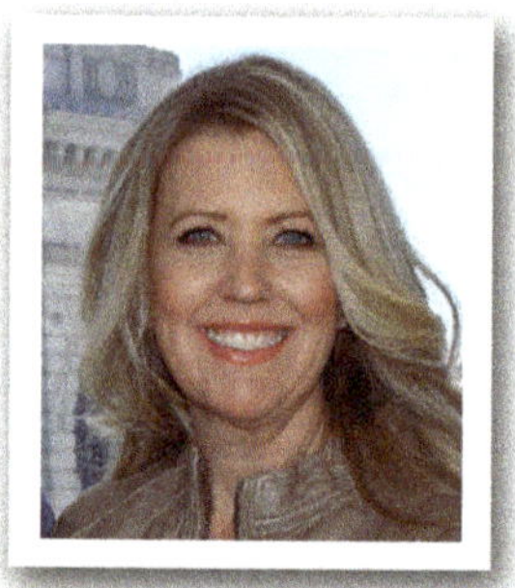

Erin Fletter

FOOD GEEK-IN-CHIEF

Erin Fletter is passionate about getting kids to not just eat, but actually crave healthy food. Erin's three enthusiastic daughters are her first round of recipe taste testers and she is never reluctant to push their culinary boundaries.

Erin loves creating hands on recipes for children that bring together fresh ingredients, global flavors, math, geography, language, nutrition, food history—and a big dash of tasty fun. Erin also writes terrible jokes about food that make everyone groan.

Erin has an extensive background in the food and wine industry and used that experience to start Sticky Fingers Cooking, a mobile and online cooking school. Sticky Fingers Cooking now has hundreds of cooking classes each week in multiple cities and has taught over 50,000 kids how to cook. Erin lives in Denver, Colorado, with her husband, three daughters, two cats and one dog; all of whom are extremely well fed.

"Wow, Chef Erin! You really write ALL of these recipes for Sticky Fingers? Good thing your food is a million times better than your jokes."

- Avery, age 6

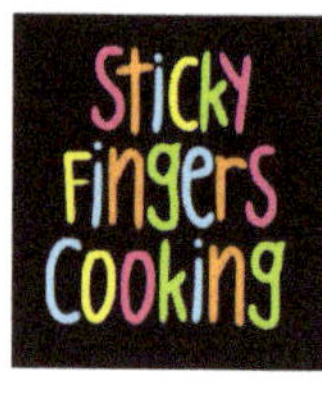

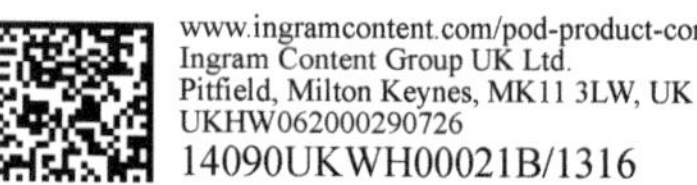

www.ingramcontent.com/pod-product-compliance
Ingram Content Group UK Ltd.
Pitfield, Milton Keynes, MK11 3LW, UK
UKHW062000290726
14090UKWH00021B/1316